BEYOND DIETING

*Psychoeducational
Interventions
for Chronically
Obese Women:
A Non-Dieting
Approach*

BRUNNER/MAZEL
EATING DISORDERS MONOGRAPH SERIES

Series Editors
PAUL E. GARFINKEL, M.D.
DAVID M. GARNER, PH.D.

EATING DISORDERS MONOGRAPH SERIES NO. 5

BEYOND DIETING

Psychoeducational Interventions for Chronically Obese Women: A Non-Dieting Approach

by

DONNA CILISKA, R.N., Ph.D.

BRUNNER/MAZEL, *Publishers* • New York

Library of Congress Cataloging-in-Publication Data
Ciliska, Donna.
  Beyond dieting : psychoeducational interventions for chronically
obese women : a non-dieting approach / by Donna Ciliska.
    p. cm.—(Brunner/Mazel eating disorders monograph series :
5)
  Includes bibliographical references.
  ISBN 0-87630-583-4
  1. Overweight women—Mental health. 2. Obesity—Psychological
aspects. 3. Body image. 4. Self-acceptance. I. Title.
II. Series.
  [DNLM: 1. Body Image. 2. Obesity—psychology. 3. Obesity—
therapy. W1 BR917D v. 5 / WD 210 C572b]
RC552.025C55 1990
616.3'98—dc20
DNLM/DLC
for Library of Congress   90-1533
                                                              CIP

Copyright © 1990 by Brunner/Mazel, Inc.

Published by
BRUNNER/MAZEL, INC.
19 Union Square West
New York, New York 10003

Manufactured in the United States of America

10 9 8 7 6 5 4 3 2 1

To our daughter, and other daughters
of the Western World:

May they grow up in a culture that accepts the whole range
of body sizes and shapes—where physical attributes are less
important than personality and abilities.

Contents

vii

Acknowledgments

No work is ever done in complete isolation from ideas and feedback from others. This monograph is no exception. Great appreciation goes to Dr. David Garner, who provided the initial enthusiasm, support, and guidance for the development and evaluation of the "Beyond Dieting" program.

I would particularly like to thank Dr. Paul Garfinkel, without whom this monograph would not have been written. His support, patience, teaching, and mentoring have been invaluable.

Thanks also go to Dr. Janet Polivy for her feedback about the program content and evaluation. In many areas, this work is an extension and/or testing of her ideas, as well as those of Dr. Peter Herman and Dr. Garner.

The program development and evaluation was done with partial financial support of fellowships from the National Health Research Development Program, the Canadian Nurses' Foundation, and the Registered Nurses' Association of Ontario. Thank you to all associated with these organizations for leaving me with the ability to concentrate on the program instead of on finances.

Finally, my friend and husband, Ian Graham, left me peaceful times to work on this monograph, calmed my anxiety about the deadlines, distracted me when I needed diversions, and gave me support and love throughout. Thanks, Ian!

Introduction

Obesity is considered a major problem in most affluent nations. Its prevalance ranges from 10% to 50% of the adult population, depending on measurement techniques and standards used (Bray, 1985). Medical complications and social stigmatization are commonly cited as the sequelae of obesity (Simopoulos & Van Itallie, 1984; Wooley & Wooley, 1979). In recent years there has been an increase in the cultural pressure on women to have a thin body (Garner, Garfinkel, Schwartz & Thompson, 1980). This goes beyond the mere avoidance of fat so that many women may equate thinness with personal worth. The pressure to be thin has also led to a proliferation of private and commercial weight loss clinics, magazine articles and books about the newest and quickest ways to lose weight, and profitable industries in diet foods and supplements. At any one time, a large proportion of the female population is either on, or planning, another diet. For young adult women, dieting has become the norm (Polivy & Herman, 1987).

Widespread cultural pressure to be thin and "anti-overweight" social prejudice, along with the experience of repeated failure at attempted weight loss, have resulted in body disparagement (Garner, Rockert, Olmsted, Johnson & Coscina, 1985) and low self-esteem in obese women (Stunkard & Mendelson, 1967; Wooley, Wooley & Dyrenforth, 1979).

Researchers have begun to question the potential untoward effects of the diet craze and have initiated critical examinations of treatments available for the overweight. In response to the question, "Should obesity be treated at all?", Wooley and Wooley (1984) have documented that treatment is mostly unsuccessful, that there is evidence for a biological control of weight and lack of clear evidence of obesity alone as a significant health risk factor, and that the stringent cultural standards of thinness for women have been accompanied by a steadily increasing incidence of severe eating disorders. They conclude that:

> It is very hard to construct a case for treating any but massive, life-endangering obesity . . . What is needed is to vigorously treat weight obsession and its manifestations: poor self and body image, disordered lifestyles, often marked by excessive or inadequate exercise, and disordered eating patterns, metabolic depression and inadequate nutrition caused by dieting. (p. 191)

But what are the alternatives to dieting for obese women who are healthy, but unhappy with their bodies? A program, called "Beyond Dieting" arose out of an attempt to respond to the Wooleys' recommendations. The group was restricted to the obese to have a more homogeneous group for evaluation of the program. Therefore, the program should not be generalized to all women, or to men. An evaluation of the program with different target groups would be useful. (The author is currently adapting and evaluating the program for younger females in the pre-teen and teen years.)

The program was developed to treat weight obsession in obese women who have made several weight-loss attempts with no long-term success. The characteristics that the Wooley's raised in the foregoing quote apply to the obese women who come to the program. They indeed have poor self-image and body image, inadequate exercise, disordered eating patterns, and inadequate nutrition. It is important to remember that not all obese women share these characteristics, but they are typical of the sample who self-select to come to the "Beyond Dieting" program.

The three basic purposes of this monograph are represented in three chapters. Chapter 1 presents the argument for the need for such a program, and the background literature for the content. Chapter 2 concerns the definition, measurement, and etiology of obesity, as well as weight regulation. Chapter 3 describes the program in enough detail for any health professional to take the information provided and conduct the program. Chapter 4 presents the evaluation of "Beyond Dieting" with the methodology and results of the randomized controlled trial with 142 participants. Chapter 5 provides general discussion of the intervention and implications for future research.

My earlier professional training led me to believe that weight loss was to be recommended to any clients who were as little as five to 10 pounds above average weight, regardless of whether they were experiencing a health problem or not. When no health problems were evident, the recommendation of weight loss was considered a preventive measure "for their own good." Informal surveys of obese women and primary care clinicians have indicated to me that this belief still guides practice in most cases. The general public gets the same message from the media, if not from their health care providers. Advertising suggests not only that extra weight is dangerous and unsightly, but also that it can be easily and painlessly lost. Simply sign a check or charge slip for the appropriate number of dollars.

But is obesity always a health risk? Is obesity always caused by overeating or underexercising? Does dieting always work? (Note: throughout this monograph, the term "dieting" means calorie re-striction for the purposes of losing weight.) Is dieting risk free? Does dieting increase self-esteem and reduce depression, or does it more often create the opposite effect? How does repeated dieting affect metabolism, glucose, and blood lipids? These are the questions addressed in Chapter 1. In many cases, an exhaustive literature review was not done, but a sampling of the two or more sides of each argument are given. The result is that it is apparent that the answers to the above questions are far less clear than some would like to believe. It seems that weight loss is not always possible or even desirable.

Chapter 3 presents detail for the psychoeducational program, with weekly objectives, group exercises, content, resources, expected reactions, and the recommended sections of background literature of Chapter 1. It is intended that any health professional could take this chapter and deliver the program. It is also expected that the content and some of the exercises would also be useful in individual counseling.

Chapter 4 reports on the evaluation of two related non-dieting interventions (education alone and a more intense psychoeducational approach). The randomized trial evaluated the effects of group interventions for clinically obese women on self-esteem, body dissatisfaction, and restrained eating. Secondary variables of interest were social adjustment, symptoms of depression, scores on bulimia and drive for thinness scales, weight, blood pressure, and serum levels of glucose and lipids. Data were collected at pretest, posttest, and six and twelve months after program completion.

Analysis indicated that the more intense psychoeducational group significantly differed from the control and educational group at posttest. Significant improvements occurred in self-esteem, with relaxation of restraint and body dissatisfaction. Means of blood pressure and weight did not change significantly. Blood values were available in numbers sufficient for analysis only in the intense group, and showed no significant changes from their beginning (normal range) levels. It is concluded that a non-dieting approach can be beneficial for the emotional health of obese women.

It is left to the individual to have an open mind in the reading of this monograph and to be able to question some long-held beliefs that form the basis of clinical practice with overweight individuals. The cultural norm may be slowly changing. There is more awareness in the general media over the past few years of some of the issues presented here—that genetics preclude some people from being skinny, that severe dieting is not healthy, that the pursuit of thinness can keep one preoccupied at the expense of more important things in life. In an ideal world of the future, programs such as "Beyond Dieting" will not be necessary. The culture will accept, equally, persons representing the whole range of body sizes and shapes without discrimination or prejudice. Caring professionals can take a leading step in promoting and supporting the cultural change.

DONNA CILISKA

BEYOND DIETING

*Psychoeducational
Interventions
for Chronically
Obese Women:
A Non-Dieting
Approach*

1

Is Dieting the Answer?

The development of ideas for this program came from the review of literature in several areas. These included definitions of the concepts of self-esteem and body image, and their theoretical underpinnings. Literature is presented here relating appearance to self-esteem, the current cultural drive for thinness, and the subsequent stigmatization of the obese. Gender and gender role differences in self-esteem are not fully examined.

Many health professionals treat the obese as though there were a standard for weight beyond which one is at high risk for the development of cardiovascular disease and Type II diabetes mellitus, and as though there were safe, effective means for all obese people to reduce weight. The basis for this belief is explored in this review, and the controversy surrounding the belief led to the inclusion of certain topics in the intervention: Is obesity a health risk? Is there an effective way to control weight? Are there any health risks involved in repeated cycles of calorie restriction followed by overeating? In order to develop these ideas, literature is included, but is not comprehensive, in the following areas: the measurement of obesity, its etiology, weight regulation, the health risks of obesity, treatments for obesity and their effectiveness, the effects of dieting, and alternative interventions to dieting for the obese.

SELF-ESTEEM, BODY IMAGE, AND THE CULTURAL DRIVE FOR THINNESS

Literature was reviewed regarding the concepts of self-esteem and body image, and the relationship of appearance to self-esteem. Our notion of standards of attractiveness are culturally determined. Thus, the cultural perspective of the current ideal of thinness in women is examined in relation to the subsequent stigmatization of those who do not meet the stringent standards of beauty and, again, the potential effect of this prejudice on the self-esteem of the obese.

Self-Esteem

A review by Wells and Marwell (1976) has shown that self-concept may be subdivided into three major domains: the specific content of the attitude toward the self (cognitive); judgment about that content relative to a standard (evaluative); and some feeling attached to that judgment (affective). Self-esteem is viewed as a subset of self-concept because it is related to the affective evaluative component. Content is considered important, but is generally thought to be secondary to the emotional tone or evaluative aspect of self-concept (Wells & Marwell, 1976, p. 59).

Many discrepant definitions of self-esteem are given by different theorists in the literature. Self-esteem has been considered to be a need (Maslow, 1954), an attitude (Coopersmith, 1967), a result of a certain level of competence (White, 1964), an index of mental health (Fitts, 1972), a moderating variable (Ziller, 1973), the purpose of all human activity (to enhance self-esteem) (Hayakawa, 1963), and an artifact, in that we cannot perceive of ourselves as objective entities (Lowe, 1961).

In keeping with the various different definitions of self-esteem, many theorists have written about the development of self-esteem from their particular theoretical framework. Freud (1923) regarded the ego in infancy and childhood to be, first, a body ego which evolves, through the process of separation-individuation, to body image. The body is, therefore, the first sense of self. Other major theorists who have considered the development of self-esteem include Adler (1929), Cooley (1956), Horney (1950), Kohut (1977) and Sullivan (1953). They have attributed the development of self-esteem to our interactions with significant others; moreover, they share the view that negative influences on the self may be minimized or reinforced by other people around us.

Cotton (1983) has synthesized several theoretical approaches in describing a developmental approach to self-esteem. During infancy, positive feelings of well-being arise from the relationship with a caregiver (usually a mother) who is responsive to the infant's needs; from the experience of one's own body which manages to effect change; and through incorporating parental behavior, personality, and the emotional milieu of the family into the sensorimotor self. The toddler develops self-esteem by differentiating the self from nonself through negativism, and by mastering motor, cognitive, and language skills. This stage involves expansion of the self through negotiation of the oral and anal stages and development of gender identity. Further skill development, parental approval, identification with parental qualities and roles, and expanded peer and teacher relationships all serve to develop self-esteem in the school-age child. Sexual identity and stronger peer relationships mark adolescence. The sense of personal identity is stronger and creates a more stable level of self-esteem.

For the purposes of this research, Rosenberg's social psychological approach (1965, 1981) to the self was used as an appropriate theoretical base for the study of obese women. Rosenberg (1965, p. 30) has defined self-esteem as a positive or negative attitude toward the self. He has developed a self-esteem scale to assess such attitudes—the extent to which individuals feel they are worthy and self-accepting, yet realistic in the sense of being aware of deficiencies and wanting to grow. While high self-esteem may connote that one thinks he or she is "good enough" or "very good," low self-esteem implies self-rejection, self-dissatisfaction, and even self-contempt.

Rosenberg (1981) expanded on earlier theorists to develop his social-psychologic approach. He further elucidated the effect on the self of interpersonal interaction, social identity, social context, and social institutions. He hypothesized that, although self-concept is located in the inner world of thought and experience, social factors play a major role in its formation so that self-concept arises:

out of social experience and interaction; it both incorporates and is influenced by the individual's location in the social structure; it is formed within institutional systems, such as the family, school, economy, church; . . . and it is affected by immediate social and environmental contexts (p. 593).

Applying this social-psychological perspective to obese women, one can see how their self-esteem would be reduced by face-to-face interaction with people whom they judge as significant and who respond to them with the general disparagement accorded most obese in our society. "We come to see ourselves as we think others see us" (Rosenberg, 1981, p. 597), imagining our appearance to the other person, imagining the judgment he or she is making of that appearance, and formulating some sort of self-feeling as a result of that judgment. Rosenberg calls this principle of self-esteem formation "reflected appraisals."

Expertise is an important basis for imputing credibility to another person. Generally, in our Western society, the medical community has seen obesity as a danger sign or in moralistic terms implying personality faults, weakness of will, or laziness in the lack of success at weight loss (Bennett & Gurin, 1982). Furthermore, the media are full of advertisements for commercial weight loss programs, diet books, and meal plans, all written and directed by the latest "expert." In summary, there are many authoritative messages in day-to-day living that give the obese woman negative "reflected appraisal."

The social context is such that interacting with people of average weight, or closer to the very thin ideal, results in a comparison that leaves obese women with even lower self-esteem. "If other people can maintain normal weight, why can't I?" This illustrates a second principle of self-esteem formation, that of "social comparison," or learning about oneself by comparison to others (Rosenberg, 1981, p. 603).

In comparison to men, or to other women, obese women are not a strong social force. That may change as the clothing and fashion industry is just beginning to address the market for better quality large-size clothing. Furthermore, the National Association to Advance Fat Acceptance (NAAFA) has recently begun to give public education, to respond to offensive advertising, to raise awareness of discrimination, and to offer support groups. However, the obese are clearly not a strong political force except for a few such small vocal groups.

Self-esteem is also affected by social identity. The "obese woman" is likely to be lower in status both in terms of income and occupation (Canning & Mayer, 1966; Elder, 1969; Larkin & Pines, 1979). This social identity element represents a basis for social evaluation that, in turn, may influence self evaluation through inner experience or "self-attribution" (Rosenberg, 1981, p. 603). In addition, obesity in women is considered deviant behavior, given the cultural norm.

The social identity element may become so important that it overwhelms all others. The obese woman may agree that she is a good wife/mother/lawyer, but discount those positive elements of her identity for the primary element of "I am fat." Self-esteem suffers when one negative part of identity is made the strongest. Rosenberg calls this aspect "psychological centrality," and he defines it as the process through which one organizes a hierarchy of what is important to the self-concept.

Self-esteem is affected by levels of satisfaction with self-concept components to which one has attributed most importance. Rosenberg (1965) found support for the principle of centrality in a study of high-school students. He found significant correlations between self-esteem and satisfaction with such self-values as honest, likable, and dependable. He later found further support for this concept in a study of adults (Rosenberg, 1979): when a quality of social identity (such as social class, income, occupational status) was judged to be very important, its effect on self-esteem was greater than if it were judged to be less important. Centrality is an important concept for this study of the obese, and will be discussed further in this review as it relates to body image and body satisfaction.

Rosenberg emphasizes the importance of addressing the personal consequences of self-esteem levels as they influence the degree to which people will lead full lives. He summarizes the literature in the area by reviewing the evidence linking self-esteem and mental illness. There are consistent relationships between low self-esteem and depression, anxiety, somatic symptoms, aggression, negative affective states, and neurotic symptoms (Rosenberg, 1981, p. 614). Robson (1988) agrees that the literature demonstrates these associations, but cautions that a causal link between self-esteem and clinical disorders has yet to be clearly established. For example, low self-esteem generally accompanies depression, and may be a causative, maintaining, or consequent factor of the depression (Robson, 1988).

Body Image

Body image is the mental picture we have of the appearance of our bodies, as well as the associated attitudes and feelings (Garner, Garfinkel, Stancer & Moldofsky, 1976). As previously stated, one's body image contributes to self-esteem and, as such, has self-perceptive and affective components, both of which may be altered as a result of development, or in reaction to specific stimuli or a set of circumstances.

The self-perceptive aspect of body image has led to the development of several tools for its measurement. These tools were developed to explore and measure body image disturbance in the obese, and were later applied to eating disorder patients. The techniques vary from distorting mirrors (Traub & Orbach, 1964), photographs (Glucksman & Hirsch, 1969) and videos of the subject (Allbeck, Hallberg & Espmark, 1976) to techniques such as "draw a person" (McCrea, Summerfield & Rosen, 1982), an image-marker method (Askevold, 1975), and a visual size estimation apparatus (Slade & Russell, 1973). Measurement of body image has resulted in widely disparate findings. Anorexics have been reported as overestimating their size (Crisp & Kalucy, 1974; Garner et al., 1976; Slade & Russell, 1973) or underestimating their size (Garner et al., 1976); normal weight women have been reported as overestimating (Crisp & Kalucy, 1974; Garner et al., 1976; Pearlson, Flournoy, Simonson & Slavney, 1981), underestimating (Garner et al., 1976), and being accurate in the measurement of their body image (Garfinkel, Moldofsky, Garner, Stancer & Coscina, 1978; Shipman & Sohlkah, 1967; Slade & Russell, 1973).

Studies of body image measurement in obesity have also led to diverse conclusions. Using a flexible mirror apparatus, Shipman and Sohlkah (1967) found that the obese substantially overestimated the widths of their lower torso. In contrast, Glucksman and Hirsch (1969) used the distorting photograph technique and found that a small sample of superobese women slightly underestimated their size. However, following the onset of a reducing diet, the subjects overestimated their size. Moreover, the degree of overestimation increased with the amount of weight lost. The subjects consistently overestimated the size of other stimuli (a model and a vase) before, during, and after weight loss, leading the authors to conclude that the obese have a general perceptual distortion leading to overestimation. Similarly, Pearlson and colleagues (1981) found that obese people attending a weight loss clinic overestimated their size (using the visual size estimation apparatus) and disliked their bodies. Neither of these factors predicted success in weight loss. Age of onset of obesity was unrelated to degree of adult obesity or to the accuracy of estimation of body width. Garner and colleagues (1976) found overestimation of body size in obese subjects. Diverse conclusions regarding body size estimation may be explained by two factors: it is possible that different techniques measure different aspects of self perception (Garner et al., 1976) and that different perceptions result from different stages of weight loss, gain, or maintenance.

Regardless of how accurate or inaccurate women are in body size estimation, women today are often reported to have negative attitudes toward their bodies. Wooley and Kearney-Cooke (1986) have hypothesized that there are two cultural changes that have influenced contemporary young women to view their bodies more negatively than at any other time in history. One is that they are the first generation of women to be exposed from infancy to the preference for thin bodies, and to be raised by mothers who are rejecting of their own bodies. Moreover, these mothers are concerned about the size of their daughters' bodies from birth. A survey of 33,000 women by "Glamour" magazine (Feeling fat, 1984) found that daughters who believed their mothers were critical of their bodies reported being more critical of their own bodies, showing poorer body image, greater use of severe dieting practices, and a higher incidence of bulimia.

> This is the heritage of anxiety and self-loathing. Women reaching maturity have not had even the respite of childhood from concerns about body size and eating, and may approach puberty with a long history of negative body image, a problem which is intensified during adolescence (Wooley & Kearney-Cooke, 1986, p. 478).

The second cultural factor affecting women's views of their bodies relates to the apparent changing role of women. Wooley and Kearney-Cooke (1986) describe the widespread ambivalence of young women about which social roles to adopt. Although they identify themselves as female, they are rejecting of the mother's social role of housewife/ mother and, with it, they reject the female body type associated with this traditional female role. They may be more accepting of the father's role of active involvement in the outside work world, and try to emulate the associated male body type. Both of these trends may have generated pressures to attain or maintain a thin physique. Other explanations for the symbolic meaning attached to the pursuit of thinness are found in Section 5.

Relationship of Satisfaction with Appearance to Self-Esteem

Dislike of one's body may have different effects on the level of self-esteem depending on the salience of body appearance to the person. To return to the issue of psychological centrality, central, rather than peripheral identity elements affect our self-esteem, that is, are seen as more salient to the self (Rosenberg, 1981, p. 607; Fleming & Watts, 1980). If appearance is considered more important to individuals than job performance and presence of good relationships, it will not matter to these individuals that they are highly skilled, in prestigious jobs, or having good relationships with co-workers, family, and friends. Their global self-esteem will be low because the judgments of their appearance are negative.

Clinical studies have described that contempt toward oneself and disturbance of body image are often seen in the obese (Glucksman, 1972; Glucksman & Hirsch, 1969; Stunkard & Mendelson, 1961). No general population studies were found in the literature which concluded that all overweight women have low self-esteem. However, there have been studies correlating body satisfaction and self-esteem that will be presented in this section. The underlying assumption of this study is that some obese women attribute their body size and appearance as salient, central factors in determining their self-esteem. Thus, their self-esteem would be lower than the self-esteem of obese women who have attributed only peripheral salience of body appearance to self-esteem. There is some support for this idea in the literature. Allen (1988), for example, conducted interviews with a small sample of women (n=37); some, but not the majority, believed that major consequences of being overweight were diminished self-image (40%) and unattractive appearance (36%). Thus, body size was not salient for most women in determining self-image or attractiveness, but was important for a significant minority.

Early research in this area, conducted by Secord and Jourard (1953), found a statistically significant relationship between self-esteem and satisfaction with one's body, which was slightly higher for females than for males. Musa and Roach (1973) later asked adolescents to rate their own appearance and that of other students in their class, and then asked students whether or not they were satisfied with how they looked. The researchers compared these ratings to a measure of self-concept. They found that there was a relationship between personal appearance and self-concept for females, but not for males. In fact, 47% of females who rated themselves equal to peers in appearance were high in ratings of self-concept, whereas 62.5% who rated themselves below their peers were low in self-concept. In a later study, attractiveness ratings were better predictors of self-concept in females, and effectiveness ratings were better predictors of self-concept in males (Lerner, Orlos & Knapp, 1976).

Satisfaction with 24 body parts has been found to be a moderate predictor of self-concept or self-esteem in college students of both sexes (Boldrick, 1983; Lerner, Karabenick & Stuart, 1973). These same two studies also tested the issue of centrality. In contrast to what may be expected from the centrality concept, ratings of subjective importance which were then weighted to body satisfaction did not significantly increase the correlation between self-esteem and body satisfaction. These findings were supported by Mahoney (1974); although two earlier studies did produce higher correlations between self-esteem and satisfaction weighted by subjective importance than correlations that were with unweighted scores of satisfaction (Rosen & Ross, 1968; Watkins & Parks, 1972).

Pliner, Chaiken and Flett (1987) found in a general population sample that females rated appearance as significantly more important to their self-esteem than did males, but had lower appearance-related self-esteem than males. However, the correlation between appearance-related self-esteem and total self-esteem was not higher for females than for males, a finding that does not support the assumption of centrality. This lack of support for the assumption of centrality was also found in a study by Shavelson and Bolus (1982). Several measures of general and specific self-concept were administered to students at two different points in time. From the data, the authors concluded that global self-concepts were not hierarchical in arrangement, but multidimensional.

Pliner and colleagues (1987) found that sex differences in concern with appearance exist across all ages from pre-adolescence to old age. Self-esteem increased with age, while importance of appearance decreased with age. In a university student sample, the same authors reported that percent overweight was significantly negatively correlated with appearance-related self-esteem for both sexes, compatible with the notion of centrality of weight to appearance.

Cash (1985) reviewed the related studies conducted between 1953 and 1983 and found that:

While objective unattractiveness is no guarantee of a poor body image, persons throughout the life-span who do perceive their own physical aesthetics negatively very often have poor self-esteem, social and heterosocial anxiety, fears of social criticism and rejection, and are less effective in their interpersonal relations (p. 199).

Although there are conflicts in the literature about the effects of subjective importance of physical attributes in predicting self-esteem, it is clear that there is, particularly for females, a positive relationship between satisfaction with appearance and self-esteem. Ratings of subjective importance of appearance do not consistently improve the correlations. One explanation is that centrality is not a consciously-mediated phenomenon—that is, the relationship between importance of appearance and self-esteem may be unconscious. In addition, Boldrick (1983) attributes the conflicting results to differences in instrumentation and analysis in the various studies. The strength of the evidence for a relationship between satisfaction with appearance and self-esteem indicates that it is important to address the potential for low self-esteem in obese women who are unhappy with their appearance, as a means of enhancing the quality of their lives.

Cultural Drive for Thinness

The literature related to the current ideal of thinness in women is reviewed because of the assumption that cultural factors are important in determining if appearance and body weight and shape are salient to self-esteem. Women are more concerned than men with body weight. There is evidence for this in the areas of dieting practices, body dissatisfaction, and eating disorders. Mazur (1986) postulates that these characteristics are a sign that women have "overadapted" to trends of feminine beauty.

Three-quarters of all female college students surveyed have dieted to control their weight (Jacobovits, Halstead, Kelley, Roe & Young, 1977). Polivy and Herman (1987) contend that among young women and adolescent girls dieting is more prevalent than non-dieting and is, thus, normative behavior. The same authors (Herman & Polivy, 1980) have reported that females score higher on a restraint scale than do males and thus are more likely to be dieting.

In an early study, Berscheid, Walster & Bohrnstedt (1973) found that 23 percent of females versus 15 percent of males surveyed were dissatisfied with their bodies. However, 45 percent of females and 55 percent of males reported being quite or extremely satisfied with their overall appearance. A survey done by a popular women's magazine (obviously not a representative sample of the general population) found that 75 percent of females rate themselves as "too fat" even though only one-quarter are actually overweight. However, 59% of the same respondents report being "moderately happy" or "very happy" with their bodies (Feeling fat, 1984). Thus, it seems women can report happiness with their bodies but still wish to be thinner.

Results of such survey responses are in accord with the findings of Garner, Olmsted & Polivy (1983). They compared the sexes on scores on the body dissatisfaction subscale of the Eating Disorder Inventory. Males reported low levels of dissatisfaction (mean=3.9) compared to females (mean=10.2). On this subscale, a higher score indicates greater body dissatisfaction.

Drewnowski and Yee (1987) found that college women were less satisfied with body shape than men. However, in a subset of men who wished to lose weight, there were no significant differences between them and the female subjects on body dissatisfaction. Fifteen percent of both males and females expressed no desire for weight change. Of the remaining subjects, 85 percent of the women wished to lose weight, whereas only 45 percent of the men wished to lose and 40 percent wished to gain. In another study, homosexual males were compared to other male groups, including those attending primary care clinics, psychology students, dance majors, and athletes (Yager, Kurtzman, Landsverk & Wiesmeier, 1988). The homosexual men scored higher on feeling fat, feeling terrified of being fat, and using diuretics, and on the Eating Disorder Inventory scales of drive for thinness, interoceptive awareness, bulimia, body dissatisfaction, maturity fears, and ineffectiveness. Thus the evidence to date indicates a much higher percentage of women and homosexual men wishing to lose weight.

Eating disorders are much more common in females. Kalucy and colleagues (1985) have calculated that only 6 percent of the anorexic patients who attended their clinic in a seven-year period were male. The prevalence of bulimia in the population varies widely depending on which diagnostic criteria are used, and depending on whether this is based on self-report or structured interviews. The prevalence of bulimic symptoms in adolescents has been identified as 9.6 percent in girls and 1.2 percent in boys (Gross & Rosen, 1988). The full syndrome of bulimia nervosa has been found to be less common (Ben-Tovim [1988] reported that 1.7 percent of females fulfilled such criteria), but the syndrome maintains the same sex ratio.

Possible explanations for the symbolic meaning attached to the pursuit of thinness in the eating disordered population include a wish to ressemble the male form as a means of succeeding in the male-dominated world (Orbach, 1978), a wish to maintain personal control in a world where an individual may feel little control (Bruch, 1978), and, in its extreme form, the return to a childlike state to avoid the responsibilities of adulthood (Crisp, 1970).

The pursuit of thinness is also related to cultural attitudes and idealization of particular body shapes for women and the association of thinness with beauty in the media. Certainly this idealization has been a fluctuating phenomenon, as witnessed by the more robust standard of beauty in Rubens' time, the slimming trend in the 1920s, and the return to popularity of the Marilyn Monroe image in the 1950s. Since the 1960s, the pendulum has swung to thinness and this time to a more extreme degree, as evidenced by Twiggy. Occasionally, the unlikely combination is proposed of thinness plus muscle, or thinness plus breasts, as models and actresses promote exercise videos and undergo breast augmentation surgery.

Assuming that Playboy magazine centerfolds and Miss America contestants represent examples of our cultural ideal of female attractiveness, Garner, Garfinkel, Schwartz and Thompson (1980) reviewed statistics of the centerfolds and contestants and compared them with population means from the Society of Actuaries. From 1959 to 1978, both the Playboy centerfolds and the contestants became significantly thinner and more "tubular," with an absolute reduction in weight, bust, and hips and an increase in height and waists. Centerfolds reduced in weight from 91 to 84 percent of average during this time, and beauty contestants reduced from 86 to 78 percent of average. Over the same period, women in North America actually gained weight, probably because of better nutrition and health care. For women in their early twenties this gain has amounted to about five pounds. The increase in average weight coupled with the idealization of thinness indicates a growing disparity between actual and "ideal" standards.

Similar data are available from Europe. Rossner (1984) has reviewed statistics of the Miss Sweden pageant and noted a significant drop in weight (from 68 to 53 kg) in the last few years (height range of 173-175 cm). Data from the Swedish National Board of Statistics indicate that means for the corresponding age group are a weight of 58 kg and height of 166 cm. When asked about their desired weight, Danish women (mean age 34, height 160 cm) have expressed a wish to be 45 kg (Schlichting, Hoilund-Carlsen & Quaade, 1981)—a weight considerably below the emaciated standard of a professional model's figure!

The reality for most women is very far from the ideal, leading them to feel as though they have failed and lack the ability to "measure up" no matter how little they eat or how much they exercise.

Stigmatization of the Obese

There is a second damaging aspect to our cultural attitudes concerning thinness—the strong prejudice against the obese (Allon, 1975). Silhouettes of the obese are described as "lazy," "stupid," "ugly," and "cheats" by children as early as age six (Staffieri, 1967). Children and adults, and the obese themselves, rate line drawings of obese children as less likable than drawings of handicapped, severely disfigured, or normal weight children (Goodman, Dornbusch, Richardson, & Hastorf, 1963; Maddox, Black, & Liederman, 1968; Richardson, Goodman, Hastorf, & Dornbusch, 1961).

A number of more recent studies have shown that judgments of peers and professionals about the mental health of subjects covary with judgments of attractiveness (Barocas & Vance, 1974; Gottheil & Joseph, 1968). In one such study, subjects rated persons on interview tapes as more disturbed and having poorer prognoses if an "unattractive" picture was attached than if there was an "attractive" one or physical anonymity (Cash, Kehr, Polyson, & Freeman, 1977). Interaction of health care providers with obese clients is also affected by the anti-fat bias. Mental health workers were asked to rate a history to which a photograph of a middle-aged woman was attached (Young & Powell, 1985). The same case was presented in every instance, but the photo was altered to be best-weight, overweight, and obese. Workers assigned more negative psychological symptoms to the obese than to the other two models. Ratings of the obese were less harsh if the health care worker was older rather than younger, male rather than female, and overweight as opposed to average weight. These findings indicate that decisions regarding severity of symptoms are affected by weight of the client, as well as by age, sex, and weight of the therapist.

It has been suggested that discrimination against obese females may be more severe than prejudice directed against obese men (Orbach, 1978; Wooley & Wooley, 1979; Wooley, Wooley, & Dyrenforth, 1979). Discrimination against the obese is manifest in lower acceptance rates at high-ranking colleges (Canning & Mayer, 1966), in a reduced likelihood of being hired for jobs in the workforce (Larkin & Pines, 1979), and in a lower possibility of movement to higher social class through marriage (Elder, 1969). In each of the above studies, the effect has been more severe for women than men. For example, Canning and Mayer (1966) noted that 23.3 percent of females and 18 percent of males graduating from high school were overweight. However, in the college freshman class, only 11.2

percent of the females were overweight, as compared to 13 percent of the males. This represented a significant difference for females but not for males. In the same study, 51.9 percent of nonobese women, versus 31.6 percent of obese women, went to college after high school graduation. There was no difference in rates for men (Canning & Mayer, 1966). However, another study of college students found no difference in severity of discrimination against the obese of either sex (Harris, Harris, & Bochner, 1982). With respect to income, a survey done for the magazine "Industry Week" showed that male executives lose an estimated $1000 per pound overweight per year ("Fat execs," 1974).

In summary, there exists a tremendous anti-fat mentality in our society that may lead to body dissatisfaction in women who try to live up to the cultural standard, and bias and discrimination against people who deviate from that ideal.

Intervention Programs for Improving Self-Esteem in Women

In North America, several community and clinical intervention programs are available to help women improve their body image and self-esteem. One of these, "Transforming Body Image" (Hutchinson, 1985), has been evaluated. Sankowsky (1981) randomly assigned 30 women with self-reported and measured negative body-cathexis to a seven-week, two-hour session of guided visuo-kinesthetic imagery or to a wait-list control group. The body Cathexis/Self Cathexis scale (Jourard & Secord, 1955) was used as a measure of body dissatisfaction and general self-esteem. Scores significantly improved in the experimental group but remained unchanged in the wait-list control group. However, the implications of the findings are limited by several issues. The study group was small and highly educated. Generalizability was further reduced by the fact that many subjects in the experimental group entered individual therapy concurrent with the study intervention. No follow-up has been reported.

Butters & Cash (1987) reported a study of college women with high levels of body-image dissatisfaction. Participants were screened from an undergraduate psychology class on the basis of low scores on a self-report instrument of attitudes to body image, self-reported weight no more than 25 percent above or below average, and lack of serious medical or current emotional problems. They were assigned to a cognitive-behavioral treatment program (n=15) of six individual sessions or a wait-list control group (n=16). The treatment group displayed improved body image, more adaptive body-image cognitions, and enhanced social self-esteem, feelings of physical fitness, and sexuality. The control group later received an abbreviated three-week treatment, with immediate effects similar to the initial treatment group, which had maintained its effect at seven-week follow-up.

One other group in Cincinnati has evaluated the effect of intensive therapy (6-8 hours per day for three and a half weeks) on bulimic women (Wooley & Kearney-Cooke, 1986). Group, individual, and family therapies were provided to 32 patients. Significant improvements were made in scores on all subscales of the Eating Disorder Inventory, the Restraint Scale, the Self and Body Cathexis Scales, and the SCL-90. This was a before-after study design with no control group comparison. Its applicability to large numbers of obese women was further reduced by the expense of the intensive therapy.

No studies were found reporting on an intervention to improve self-esteem or body dissatisfaction in obese women.

2

Obesity: Definition, Measurement, Etiology, and Attempts at Regulation

In the literature, "overweight" and "obesity" are often used inter-changeably, or without specifying if the categorization is based on actual weight, a particular percent over a matched population standard or an ideal standard, body mass index, skin fold measurements, or an estimate of percent body fat. Also, techniques for measuring body weight or proportion of fat differ from study to study. Consequently, estimates of the prevalence of obesity range from 10 to 50 percent or more of the adult population (Bray, 1985).

The literature related to definitions of obesity was explored in order to establish a definition for the evaluation component of this program. Weight is commonly expressed as a percent of a standard such as the "ideal" of the Metropolitan Life Tables, or average of the Health and Welfare (Canada) tables. Obesity has been defined as any weight at or above 115 percent of ideal (Schachter, 1981), and at the other end of the spectrum, greater than 25 percent above average (Garner et al., 1976). Obesity for this project was defined as 20 percent above average. A definition of obesity as a percent of average is frequently used in studies as it is convenient and sensitive to change. However, weight may increase for reasons other than fat deposition, such as increased muscle mass in response to exercise. Therefore, percent of average weight is not a useful definition when studying effects of exercise.

21

Today, most people adhere to a model of obesity that emphasizes its heterogeneous and multidimensional nature. There are environmental, behavioral, genetic, physiological, and socioeconomic variables influencing the development and/or maintenance of obesity. These factors will be considered either in this section or under the "Weight Regulation" section that follows.

Simply, obesity is caused by the ingestion of too many calories and/or utilization of too little energy. No totally successful attempt has been made to classify etiologies of human obesities. However, Sclafani (1984) has classified 50 different animal models of obesity into neural, endocrine, pharmacological, nutritional, environmental, seasonal, genetic, viral, and idiopathic categories. He concludes that the many different types of animal obesities indicate that no single type can serve as a general model of human obesity.

There are now several examples of genetically obese animals used in research (Sclafani, 1984). However, no "obesity" gene has been identified as yet in humans. Nevertheless, several studies have shown evidence of genetic determination of obesity in humans (i.e., Borjeson, 1976; Brook, Huntley & Slack, 1975; Feinleib et al., 1977). From a genetic epidemiologic approach, Bouchard (1986) has concluded that the mean genetic contribution to percent body fat is 20 to 25 percent of the total variance.

Similarly, Stunkard has reported the results of two relevant studies. In a study of 1974 monozygotic and 2097 dizygotic male twin pairs followed up 25 years after an assessment for induction into the army (Stunkard, Foch & Hrubec, 1986), concordance rates for different degrees of overweight were twice as high for monozygotic twins as for dizygotic twins. The investigators estimated a high heritability for height, weight, and Body Mass Index (BMI) at age 20 years (0.80, 0.78 and 0.77 respectively) and at 25-year follow-up (0.80, 0.81 and 0.84). In a study of 540 Danish adults who had been adopted as very young children, (Stunkard, Sorenson et al., 1986), a strong positive relationship was reported between weight classification of adult adoptees and BMI in biological parents, but no relationship was found between adoptees and adoptive parents.

Stunkard and colleagues thus concluded that genetic influences are important in determining human fatness in adults, whereas family environment alone has no apparent effect.

Ravussin et al. (1988) studied metabolic rate of southwestern American Indians and found subjects with low 24-hour energy expenditure (measured in a respiratory chamber) had a fourfold increased risk of gaining considerable weight at two-year follow up. The observed metabolic deficiency was not sufficient, alone, to account for the degree of weight gain. This implied that an increase in food intake also contributed to the new weight level. This study also indicated that a low rate of energy expenditure was a familial trait and contributed to the aggregation of obesity in families. The three foregoing studies indicate that obesity has a high genetic or heritability factor.

Psychodynamic theories have often assumed that obesity is a psychoneurotic or psychosomatic disorder (Kaplan & Kaplan, 1957). Unconscious conflicts arising from disruptions in personality development are thought to lead to overeating, or overeating is thought to be a response to emotional distress as anxiety and depression (McReynolds, 1982). Bruch (1973) described overeating and obesity as related to developmental or reactive issues. Obesity that followed the experience of trauma was labeled by her as "reactive." In contrast, she described developmental obesity and anorexia nervosa as a result of faulty hunger awareness—hunger and satiety are not innately identifiable but subject to learning. Disturbances of hunger awareness develop from inaccuracies in the reciprocal feedback patterns in mother-infant interactions. Thus, Bruch described developmental obesity in children whose mothers superimposed their own concept of need on the child.

There are no consistent findings in the literature supporting an association between psychological disturbance and obesity in non-clinical populations. Studies of the obese from a psychiatric perspective have found them to be a heterogeneous group, with a distribution of psychiatric illness that occurs in the general population (McReynolds, 1982; Stunkard, 1976). Nevertheless, some obese people may use their obese state in a psychopathological manner to distance from or exercise power over others.

Socioeconomic factors affect the prevalence of obesity. In the United States, women below the poverty line have a much higher prevalence of obesity at all ages above 25 years: 5 percent of women in the upper socioeconomic status group, 16 percent of middle status, and fully 30 percent in lower status groups are considered obese. For men, 32 percent of the lower status group are obese compared with 16 percent in the upper group (Goldblatt, Moore, & Stunkard, 1965). The 1985 Canada Fitness Survey found that 17 percent of adult females who earn less than $10,000 per year had a BMI in excess of 28.6 (considered too high) whereas only 5 percent of adult females who earn more than $35,000 per year were in this category. For men, 14 percent who earn less than $10,000 had a BMI less than 20.1 (considered too low) and only 2 percent of males who earn more than 35,000 were in this category. This survey also found that a higher percent of men are overweight or obese at all age levels, but women are more likely to seek weight loss.

WEIGHT REGULATION

The literature on weight regulation was reviewed to challenge the popular notion that weight can easily be gained or lost depending on change in caloric balance. There is considerable evidence that body weight can be maintained despite marked variations in food intake (Booth, 1980; Keesey, 1980; Miller, 1982; Newsholme, 1982; Rothwell & Stock, 1983).

Adaptations to Excess Energy Intake

Normal subjects fattened by overeating require more energy in relation to their body surface for maintenance of the obese state than they require at their natural weight, and more than the spontaneously obese (Sims, Danforth, Horton et al., 1973). This suggests that subjects have a natural tendency to "burn-off" excess food rather than to store it. The idea that the body can adapt to overnutrition by disposing of excess energy as heat was originally called "Luxusconsumption" (Neumann, 1902). It has also been called the "specific dynamic action of food," and "non-shivering thermogenesis," and is now referred to as "diet-induced thermogenesis" (DIT).

One possible mechanism for such increased heat production is through thermogenesis in brown fat. Evidence exists for the thermoregulatory functioning of brown adipose tissue (BAT) in the newborn of several species, including rats and humans (Hervey & Tobin, 1983). However, the literature abounds with contradictions about the role of brown fat thermogenesis. One of the strongest cases against brown fat thermogenesis in adults comes from the same authors (Hervey & Tobin, 1983) who believe brown adipose cells are reduced to nil or only trace numbers in humans after one year of age; the excess energy supposedly "burned off" may merely be the result of error in measurement of food intake or metabolic rate.

Others are not so quick to dismiss brown fat activity and its role in weight regulation. For example, Rothwell and Stock (1983) believe there is some histological and thermographic evidence to suggest humans retain some functional BAT, but that direct confirmation of BAT could be exceptionally difficult. They have calculated that as little as 40-50 gm of BAT could, if maximally stimulated, make the difference between maintaining a constant body weight or gaining at the rate of 20 kg/year.

Another possible mechanism for thermogenesis is an increase in the rate of substrate cycling, that is, an increased rate of hydrolysis of adenosinetriphosphate to adenosinediphosphate and phosphate. The rate of these cycles may be increased by stress, exercise, and overfeeding in normal weight adults (Newsholme, 1982).

Any of these mechanisms may be impaired in the obese, contributing to the initiation and/or maintenance of the condition. However, work that provides empirical evidence for such mechanisms is, at present, lacking.

Adaptations to Inadequate Energy Intake

When caloric intake falls below normal values, there is an initial drop in weight followed by a marked decrease in the rate of energy expenditure. The basal metabolic rate is depressed (Keys et al., 1950). Consequently, the number of calories required just for weight maintenance drops. A return to normal levels of food intake is sufficient to promote rapid weight gain (Booth, 1980).

Donahoe and colleagues (1984) studied 10 women, first to get a baseline, then to examine metabolic rates following a period of restricted intake. They asked the participants to restrict their daily intake to 800 kcals for two weeks. By self report, mean intake was 1100 kcals for the next four weeks. Six weeks of dietary restriction lowered the resting metabolic rate by an amount almost double what would have been expected on the basis of the resulting weight loss. This confirms that energy-conserving adaptations do occur during periods of caloric restriction, and suggests an explanation for the decline in weight loss that typically occurs shortly after the initiation of a reducing program.

In a more carefully controlled study, Bray (1969) admitted obese patients to a hospital ward devoted to studying metabolism. He reduced their intake from 3500 kcals to 450 kcals/day for 24 days. Oxygen consumption declined by more than 17 percent even though weight loss was quite small (less than 3 percent). The decrease in energy expenditure greatly exceeded actual loss of tissue.

Geissler, Miller and Shah (1987) matched 16 "post-obese" (who were at or near target weight for at least six months) with 16 lean controls and measured their metabolic rates in a room respirometer. The "post-obese" had metabolic rates about 15 percent lower than controls at sleep, exercise, or sedentary activity. Their caloric intake was 70 percent of controls. As the "post-obese" regained weight, metabolic rate rose to a level equal to or greater than normals, to a point where the obese weight could be maintained on a caloric intake similar to the intake needed just for weight maintenance of the lean controls. Thus the same number of calories maintains the obese at a high weight as maintains the lean at a normal one.

Each of these studies supports the notion that the body defends a weight that is natural for the individual even if it is not statistically "normal."

"Set-Point"

Because of these adaptations to excess and inadequate energy intake, it has been postulated that a predisposition to obesity or leanness is genetically determined (Miller, 1982), and the organism resists displacement from a body weight "set-point" by adjusting the rate of energy expenditure (Booth, 1980).

Keesey (1980) has argued that although variability in weight within a species is evidence against a set-point, weight is very stable over an extended period of time within an individual. The fact that stability is maintained under differing environmental and physiological conditions supports the view that body weight, like body temperature or total body water, is regulated around some reference level or set-point. This set-point is defended by controlling both the rate of ingestion and the rate of energy expenditure.

In his review of both the animal and human literature, Keesey (1986) has questioned the etiology of obesity, asking whether it is caused by: 1) an eating disorder where the obese lack appropriate control over food intake, 2) a failure in energy expenditure mechanisms in the body such as reduced diet-induced thermogenesis, or 3) a regulation of body weight around an elevated set-point. He has concluded that there are two main types of obesity.

One type of obesity is that of regulatory failure in which there is a period of overeating. In this type, the conventional therapies of dieting, behavior modification, and physical activity are effective. Certainly, some people gain adiposity by overeating and remain overweight and above their set-point through a high caloric intake. Keesey has suggested that these patients could lose weight by creating an energy deficit for a period of time, without incurring adverse metabolic adaptations until they reached their set-point weight.

The other type of obesity involves physiological regulation around an elevated set-point. In this situation, energy-conserving mechanisms render the above therapies less effective and very difficult to sustain for a lifetime. Subjects may be successful in short-term weight loss through dieting, but as the body becomes more efficient at energy conservation, the individual's weight reaches a plateau. Rapid weight gain occurs when energy intake returns to normal. Keesey does not estimate what proportion of the obese population is regulating about a high set-point. However, it is this group that is engaged in a continuous, rigorous struggle to keep from gaining weight on a very low energy intake. Differentiation between these two types could be accomplished by observing the effects of weight gain or loss on resting metabolic rate, or by studying the heat increment of a meal to reveal the presence or absence of physiological adjustment.

There has been no direct confirmation of a body weight set-point and there are several arguments against it (Booth, 1980): 1) people vary sometimes by many pounds between weighings even when they are not "watching" their energy balance; 2) average adult weight is not constant but gradually increases until old age; 3) adult steady average weight may be markedly higher or lower in different social or physical environments; 4) belief in a physiological set-point may create a cognitive set-point which may become antitherapeutic in that patients with related health problems will be discouraged from attempting weight loss.

Some of the above arguments are related to the use of the term. Mrosovsky and Powley (1977) reviewed the literature to find that "set-point" is used as a description of experimental findings, as reflecting adaptive or biological functions of fat, and finally, as implying a particular kind of control system with a reference signal. They have concluded that the term can be valuable with any of these meanings, as long as one is clear about which definition is utilized. Certainly, the different meanings contribute to confusion and debates related to the concept.

In summary, obesity is a condition characterized by excess of adipose tissue that is thought to have complex and multiple etiologies including genetic, environmental, behavioral, and physiological factors.

OBESITY AS A HEALTH RISK FACTOR

The literature was reviewed relative to the health risks of obesity, not to be exhaustive, but to answer these questions: Are there any instances in which an obese person should try to maintain, instead of trying to lose weight? Is it ethical for a health professional to suggest that an obese person give up dieting attempts? Massive obesity certainly affects the quality of life, if not the length of life, in terms of emotional stress, mobility, and respiratory and circulatory functioning. However, debate is evident in the literature as to the extent of risk involved in being less than 100 percent above ideal weight. Is obesity an independent risk factor, or merely an associated factor to other risk factors? Does obesity cause poor health or just statistically covary with some diagnoses?

The following comparison of literature on mortality and morbidity outcomes related to obesity is hampered by differences in definitions of obesity used, methods of sample selection, study time frame, outcomes, and presence of confounding variables.

Morbidity

MacMahon et al. (1987) reviewed population and prospective studies in relation to obesity and hypertension. They found that, in most studies, blood pressure increased linearly with increasing body weight and BMI. However, in the Framingham study, this effect was greater in the younger than in older populations (Hubert et al., 1983). They estimated one-third of all hypertension is attributable to obesity, and obesity and hypertension increase the risk of cardiovascular disease. However, they cautioned that it is uncertain if risks associated with hypertension and the benefits of treatment are as great in obese as in lean hypertensives.

Contradictory evidence was found in the Tecumseh study (Epstein et al., 1965) of a whole population. Overall correlations between blood pressure and weight were insignificant (for systolic pressure and weight, $r=0.253$, diastolic pressure and weight, $r=0.259$). More dramatically, 6,966 family practice patients were assessed for five-year rates of cardiovascular events. A multivariate analysis controlling for age, sex, smoking, drinking, and severity of hypertension showed obese hypertensives to have only 0.58 the risk of cardiovascular event compared to nonobese hypertensives. Inaccurate blood pressure measurement in the obese was ruled out as an explanation. When males were subdivided into obese, normal, and underweight categories, a highly significant linear trend was found, with the highest rate of cardiovascular event present among the underweight. The authors concluded that perhaps hypertension associated with obesity runs a more benign course (Bass, Buck & Donner, 1985).

It may be that some morbidity is due to chronic dieting rather than to to obesity itself. Animal evidence suggests hypertension associated with obesity may be a result of dieting. Animals repeatedly starved to lose 20 percent or more of their weight and then refed, develop high blood pressure, undergo damage to their blood vessels, and develop cardiovascular disease (Ernsberger & Haskew, 1987).

The American Cancer Society longitudinal study of 750,000 people has reported that as weight increases, digestive system diseases and cancer increase (colorectal and prostatic for men; breast, cervix, endometrium, uterus, and ovary for women) (Lew & Garfinkel, 1979). Bray's review (1985) further documents obesity-related morbidity to be hyperinsulinemia, hyperlipidemia, impaired glucose tolerance, diabetes mellitus, and gallbladder disease.

Mortality

The National Institutes of Health Consensus Development Conference (1985) has concluded that obesity is associated with increased morbidity and mortality. The American Cancer Society study supports the idea that as weight increases, mortality from cardiovascular disease and diabetes mellitus increases, but not until Body Mass Index (BMI=weight in kilograms/square of height in meters) reaches 25 (Lew & Garfinkel, 1979). Bray (1978) has further concluded that significant increases in mortality do not appear until the BMI rises to 30 or more.

Several researchers have reviewed the same longitudinal population studies and come to different conclusions about mortality risk associated with obesity. Simopoulos and Van Itallie (1984) have concluded that overweight persons die sooner than average weight persons, and that obesity is an independent predictor of cardiovascular disease. In the Framingham study, 26-year data have detected ischemic heart disease in subjects of severe obesity of long duration (Hubert et al., 1983). Manson and colleagues (1987) have concluded the same studies underestimate the impact of obesity on mortality and that lowest mortality rates actually occur at weights 10 percent below average.

However, there are suggestions in the literature that obesity may not be a separate risk factor but merely an association with other risk factors (Mayer, 1966). Brunzell (1984) has argued that though morbidity is increased for cardiovascular risk factors, mortality is not. He hypothesized that a significant portion of the risk of obesity of coronary artery disease is mediated through specific familial disorders that are associated with both obesity and premature coronary artery disease, but is not a result of obesity alone. Andres (1980), and Ernsberger and Haskew (1987) have reviewed the major population studies of obesity and mortality and have found that they fail to show that obesity leads to any greater mortality risk. Andres (1980) even suggests moderate obesity may be associated with some benefits.

Researchers are now describing a subgroup of the obese that accounts for some of the discrepancies in findings of mortality and morbidity. Distribution of obesity on the body may be important. Prospective studies have shown abdominal obesity is a risk factor for cardiovascular disease independent of BMI or degree of obesity (Krotkiewski et al., 1983; Lapidus et al., 1984; Larrson et al., 1984). Abdominal obesity is also associated with hyperinsulinemia, glucose intolerance, and hypertriglyceridemia (Kissebah et al., 1982; Krotkiewski et al., 1983). This pattern of "android" fat distribution is much more common in men than in women. Yet women far outnumber men in their concern about weight and in attendance at commercial and clinical weight loss programs.

It may be argued that the obese should never give up trying to lose weight because of the health risks involved in obesity. However, even if one accepts that for some obese subgroups there are risk factors, does weight loss reduce those risks? There are few studies in this area because dropout rates are very high in weight loss programs and maintenance of weight loss is so poor. MacMahon's review (1987) has concluded that weight reduction lowers blood pressure but is only a short-term measure for most people since maintenance is unlikely. Similarly, Haynes (1986) has concluded that weight loss for overweight hypertensives offers limited benefit and delays the implementation of more effective therapy.

Mental Health Risks

Given the societal pressure to be thin and discrimination against deviance from this ideal, it is remarkable that the obese show no greater psychopathology than the nonobese in general population studies (Moore, Stunkard & Srole, 1962; Silverstone, 1968). In fact, the obese have shown some advantages over the nonobese in lower levels of depression and anxiety (Crisp & McGuiness, 1976; Stewart & Brobek, 1983). Wadden and Stunkard (1985) have reviewed 30 studies in clinical populations and concluded that obese patients report no greater degree of psychological disturbance than the non-obese on objective tests or psychiatric interview: "These are important findings because they refute the long-standing belief that overweight persons suffer from serious emotional disturbances" (p. 1064).

Although evidence from controlled studies has indicated that the obese do not display greater emotional disturbance in most areas of functioning than the nonobese, they demonstrate disparagement related to their own body. Using the Body Dissatisfaction subscale of the Eating Disorder Inventory, obese women (N=44) have scored significantly higher (X= 21.1, p<0.001) than subjects with Anorexia Nervosa (N=113, X=17.4), those recovered from Anorexia Nervosa

(N=17, X=6.3, p<0.0001), a female comparison group (N=577, X=10.2, p<0.001), or a male comparison group (N=166, X=3.9, p<0.001) (Garner, Olmsted & Polivy, 1983). This supports earlier work by Stunkard and his colleagues who found that the obese describe themselves as "loathsome," "slobs," and "pigs," feel self-conscious, and believe others view them with hostility and contempt. (Stunkard & Burt, 1967; Stunkard & Mendelson, 1961, 1967).

In summary, the literature indicates obesity is not a risk factor for the development of major psychological disturbance nor a result of such a disturbance. Even if one accepts that obesity alone is a risk factor for physical disease, the lack of success in treating the condition is discouraging. Therefore, it may be better to normalize eating and to reduce the body disparagement and low self-esteem resulting from repeated failure at weight loss attempts than to continue the unsuccessful and stressful attempts to diet. The success of such an intervention has potential benefit for a large number of adult women.

ATTEMPTED TREATMENTS OF OBESITY AND OUTCOMES

Thousands of "cures" exist for obesity. For the individualist who prefers to "do it on her own," there are innumerable magazine articles, books, and videos for advice and plans. If help is sought, one could go to a physician, nurse, nutritionist, psychologist, health educator, fitness consultant, or any number of lay counselors, who might provide drugs, surgery, diet and exercise plans, behavior modification, and individual or group support. Are they effective?

Review of the weight loss literature is difficult due to several methodological issues. Different criteria for defining obesity (as stated in this introduction) make the study samples inconsistent. That is, studies using only moderately obese have been compared to studies using mildly overweight or severely obese subjects. Similarly, different criteria have been used for success. Drop-out rates have tended to be very high and have been handled in different ways in the analyses. In addition, follow-up has been very short, with few studies reporting outcomes even at one year. Examples, rather than an exhaustive review of different programs, are presented in the following.

Surgery, such as gastric stapling, is most effective and is reserved for morbid obesity (above 100 percent over ideal weight) (Stunkard, 1984). The morbidly obese have not only lost weight following surgery but also experienced fewer emotional reactions usually associated with dieting (depression, anxiety, and body-image disparagement), felt more elated and self-confident (Halmi, Stunkard & Mason, 1980), felt sated with less food, and changed food choices by reducing frequency of intake of high-density fat and carbohydrates (Halmi et al., 1981). In a review of jejunoileal bypass surgery, overall patient satisfaction with the psychosocial outcomes of surgery was high in spite of complications which included a 4 percent mortality rate, 25 percent reversal rate, and 33 percent readmission rate for complications (McFarland, Gazet & Pilkington, 1985). Stunkard and colleagues found that complications were reduced with gastric stapling; only 7 percent of patients experienced severe complications. Mean weight loss was 43 kg, which constituted a loss of 66 percent of excess weight. However, about two-thirds reported nausea, vomiting, and abdominal pain after eating for periods up to several months following surgery (Stunkard, Stinnet & Smoller, 1986).

Other treatments for the morbidly obese have been described. For example, Kaufman (1986) has found that gastric balloon treatment resulted in 0.75-1.3 kg weight loss per week. However, when a control group received the same dietary and behavior treatment, balloon-treated patients had a mean weekly weight loss of only 200g per week more than the control. Little long-term follow-up has been done to determine maintenance after balloon removal. In another study (McFarland et al., 1987) 12 obese were treated with a gastric balloon for 12 to 24 months. They lost up to 21 kg over the first three months, weight plateaued for a period, then they regained. At one year, only one patient maintained weight loss. The authors concluded that gastric balloons are of no value in the treatment of weight loss.

Another suggested treatment, suction-assisted lipectomy, is not effective for generalized obesity. It has been recommended for use as cosmetic surgery for people of normal weight who want, for example, to remove some fat from their thighs, upper arm, or neck (Ersek et al., 1986).

For the mild or moderately obese, anorectic pharmacologic agents such as fenfluramine are effective in inducing weight loss. However, weight is quickly restored to the original level when the medication is stopped (Stunkard, 1984). One study compared behavior modification alone, medication alone, and combined treatment. After one year, the behavior modification group was most successful at maintenance of weight loss (Stunkard & Penick, 1979).

A number of other agents are currently under review, such as ephedrine/methylxanthine derivatives which cause a significant increase in 24-hour energy expenditure in the obese but not in lean subjects (Dulloo & Miller, 1986). In a randomized trial of femoxetine (methyl phenypiperidine) with obese patients (Bitsch & Skrumsager, 1987), both the drug group and the placebo group were placed on 1200-1600 kcal of intake per week for 16 weeks. There was no significant difference in weight loss between groups. The antidepressant fluoxetine (bezenepropanamine) has an anorectic effect on humans and has been shown to enhance weight loss in non-depressed subjects in an eight-week treatment trial (Ferguson & Feighner, 1987).

In addition to appetite suppressants, other pharmacologic research involves drugs that suppress food intake and inhibit gastric emptying (chlorocitric acid and cholecystokinin), drugs that reduce bioavailability of dietary carbohydrate (acarbose) or lipid (tetrahydrolipsin), and other thermogenic drugs (Sullivan, 1986). These drugs are in very early stages of investigation with animals or have had very short-term trials with humans without follow-up. At the present time, there are no effective pharmacologic agents that allow clinically significant weight loss and maintenance.

Behavioral therapists have attempted to intervene in obesity by reducing meal size, bite size, speed of ingestion, and type of food. These attempts have been based on the assumption that the obese eat more food, more frequently, and at higher speed than average weight individuals. Studies done in fast food restaurants (Coll, Meyers & Stunkard, 1979; Stunkard, Coll, Lindquist, & Meyers, 1980), naturalistic settings (Mahoney, 1975), or self-report (Kisseleff, Jordan & Levitz, 1978) have demonstrated that this is not the case. There is no characteristic eating style in the obese. In addition, behavioral therapy has not been as powerful as hoped in that self-applied behavioral techniques are extinguished when therapist contact is ended (Foreyt, Goodrick & Gotto, 1981). Anorectic drugs have been combined with behavior therapy with no improvement in results (Craighead, 1984).

Despite these limitations, Wing and Jeffrey (1979) have analyzed all available studies of outpatient treatment of obesity between 1966 and 1977. Treatments included anorectic drugs, HCG and thyroid hormones, exercise, diets, and behavior therapy. Initial weight loss was similar across all treatment modalities. Most patients showed weight gain after termination of the program. This happened significantly less frequently in the behavior therapy group. However, after one year, even subjects in the behavior therapy group showed they had regained all the lost weight, or maintained only minimal weight loss.

Long-term results have not improved much in the 10 years since Wing and Jeffrey's review (1979). Stalonas, Perri and Kerzner (1984) followed subjects five years after a behavioral treatment program and found the average subject was slightly heavier at follow-up than at pretreatment. Brownell and Wadden (1986) compared controlled trials of behavior therapy for obesity completed before and during 1974, during 1978 and 1984. In 1984, the average length of treatment was 13 weeks with a weight loss of 15 pounds. At follow-up, the average weight loss was 9.8 pounds at 58 weeks. This was a clinically insignificant weight loss, since the average subject was 48 percent overweight. The authors, however, were optimistic in that this represented substantial improvement over previous results. They attributed their modest success to the combination of behavior modification, cognitive change, social support, exercise, and nutrition.

Self-help and commercial weight loss groups have reported very positive results but have not been exposed to rigorous evaluation. Those few that have been studied are hard to evaluate due to very high drop-out rates—67 percent in one self-help group (Levitz & Stunkard, 1974) and 70 percent in a commercial program (Volkmar, Stunkard, Woolston & Bailey, 1981).

The most optimistic work has been the combination of very low calorie diets and behavior therapy. Clinically significant weight losses (mean 42.5 pounds) were achieved with an average regain at one year of about one-third of the weight lost, resulting in a net loss of 28 pounds (Brownell & Wadden, 1986). The same authors have hypothesized that maintenance can be further improved in future clinical trials through exercise, social support, and behavior modification (with emphasis on relapse training) (Brownell & Wadden, 1986).

Currently, there are no consistent personality factors associated with success in the treatment phase of weight loss. There is some evidence that those who exercise and have social support are more likely to lose weight (Brownell, 1984). In searching for predictors of maintenance, Snow and Harris (1985) compared, at one year after at least 20-pound weight loss, 72 maintainers versus 103 regainers. Maintainers were more likely to be male, younger, better educated, and to have weighed less as teens and adults, and have had fewer overweight sisters and friends. Marston and Criss (1984) followed 47 formerly overweight persons by mailed questionnaire for one year. Fifty-eight percent limited their regain to less than 20 percent of the amount of weight lost. Maintainers were more likely to exercise several times per week and less likely to eat for emotional reasons.

In the obese, exercise has not shown consistent benefit in reducing weight, changing body composition to lean body mass, or having a prolonged thermogenic effect beyond the activity (Pacy, Webster & Garrow, 1986). However, exercise should be part of any intervention program for the obese for its other benefits. These include lower insulin levels, improved blood profiles of glucose and lipids,

(Bjorntorp, 1976; Brownell & Stunkard, 1980), and improved mood and self-esteem (Folkins & Sime, 1981).

With regard to outcomes of treatment, little has changed since Stunkard's (1958) conclusion: "Most obese people do not enter treatment for obesity. Of those who do enter, most will not remain. Of those who remain, most will not lose weight. Of those who lose weight, most will regain it."

One cautiously optimistic report comes from Schachter (1981). In a retrospective study using self-report, he conducted open-ended interviews with a nongeneralizable convenience sample of 161 people about their attempts at self-cure for smoking and overweight. Of the group with a history of obesity who had actively tried to lose weight (N=40), 62.5 percent were categorized as successful cures. They lost an average of 34.7 pounds and maintained the weight loss for an average of 11.2 years. Schachter has concluded that the rate of self-cure is considerably higher than anything reported in the therapeutic literature, and can be explained in terms of self-selection—only the most difficult cases seek help. Thus, perhaps people can and do lose weight, and maintain the weight loss on their own. The dismal results of interventions reported in the literature may reflect the resistant population who avail themselves of treatment.

EFFECTS OF DIETING

Dieting is not risk-free. In addition to inadequate nutrition and its consequences, dieting has been implicated in the development of depression, irritability, fatigue, weakness, social withdrawal, loss of sexual drive, "semistarvation neuroses" (Glucksman, 1972), and sudden death from cardiac arrhythmias (Van Itallie & Yang, 1984).

Early evidence of negative reactions to dieting came from the Keys et al. study (1950) where one-quarter of the normal-weight volunteers experienced depression, apathy, loss of sex drive, and preoccupation with food on semistarvation diets.

In one study of overweight, more than half of the participants involved in weight loss had adverse emotional reactions (Stunkard,

1957). Such disturbances have been found to be intensified among morbidly obese dieters (Halmi, Stunkard & Mason, 1980). Nutzinger, Cayiroglu, Sachs and Zapotoczky (1985) reported a marked increase in depressive symptoms in the obese after four weeks of dieting, as measured by a self-report scale (Zung) and a clinician interview (Hamilton Depression Scale). However, subjects chosen had mild levels of depression at entry to the study. Evidence for long-term depression was unavailable as an antidepressant was given at the time. The medication reduced depressive symptoms below baseline and, in the long term, had a positive effect on weight loss.

The evidence supporting adverse consequences to dieting and weight loss is inconsistent, with some studies reporting improved psychological functioning or no change in this dimension following either dieting (Wing, Epstein, Marcus & Kupfer, 1984) or gastric surgery (Stunkard, Stinnet & Smoller, 1986). Desirable changes following dieting include decreased anxiety, decreased depression (Wadden, Stunkard & Smoller, 1986), and decreased general emotional distress (Linet & Metzler, 1981), as well as increased self-esteem (Crumpton, Wine & Groot, 1966). Post-surgical changes have included improved mood and self-esteem (Solow, Silverfarb & Swift, 1974; Stunkard, Stinnet & Smoller, 1986).

The apparent inconsistencies are probably due to different methodologies in the measurement of adverse reactions. In an invited review of dieting and depression, Smoller, Wadden and Stunkard (1987) have found that studies using instruments such as questionnaires, inventories, or checklists have reported either no change or improvement in emotional reactions. Studies using assessments such as open-ended psychiatric interviews have reported untoward emotional reactions. Psychiatric interview is usually considered the gold standard, as self-report instruments are open to denial and response bias. Inconsistencies could also result from differences in methods used to lose weight, measurement times, and definitions of overweight and obesity that affect inclusion of subjects, length of caloric restriction, degree of weight loss (Glucksman, 1972), speed of weight loss (Taylor, Ferguson & Reading, 1978), and length of follow-up.

Herman, Polivy and colleagues have developed and are continuing to test the concept of restraint. They have shown that individuals who are relatively food deprived (that is, dieting or "restrained") can be disinhibited in their eating, so that they eat more than unrestrained people after a high-calorie preload (Herman & Mack, 1975; Hibscher & Herman, 1977), after alcohol consumption (Polivy & Herman, 1976), and when anxious (Herman & Polivy, 1975). The disinhibitor temporarily ruins the diet and leads to overeating. Most dieters do not maintain uninterrupted dieting, but have alternating periods of restraint and overeating, which do not allow for significant weight loss or maintenance, nor do they result in weight gain at a steady rate.

The boundary model of eating (Herman & Polivy, 1984) postulates that there is a "zone of biological indifference" in which the person is neither famished nor full when eating, and which can be affected by non-physiological cues. Restrained eaters cognitively create a diet boundary that reduces the amount of food allowed and lowers the likelihood of experiencing satiety. However, the satiety level may be higher in restrained eaters once the diet barrier is broken (Polivy, Herman, Olmsted & Jazwinski, 1984). Chronic dieters may become relatively insensitive to internal cues of hunger, mislabel them, or learn to ignore them.

Chronically restrained eating also leads to heightened external cue responsiveness, overwhelming hunger, and faltering control over food intake (Herman & Polivy, 1980), and may be a risk factor in the development of bulimia (Polivy & Herman, 1985; Garner et al., 1985). Two studies have documented a co-relationship of dieting with binge eating (Casper et al., 1980; Pyle, Mitchell & Ekert, 1981). In fact, surveys report 80-88 percent of bulimic patients were trying to lose weight at the time of their initial binge-purge episode (Fairburn & Cooper, 1982; Pyle, Mitchell & Eckert, 1981).

Telch and colleagues (1988) conducted a descriptive study of the relationship between overweight and binge eating. They found binge eating becomes significantly more prevalent as the degree of obesity increases. Subjects were grouped according to BMI quartile ranks.

At BMI quartiles of 23-25, 25-28, 28-31, and 31-42, the prevalence of DSM-III bulimics was found to be 4.8 %, 10%, 15%, and 40% respectively. However, these researchers have acknowledged that their study has not answered the question of causality. Does excessive dieting associated with being overweight lead to binge eating, which in turn increases caloric intake and weight gain? Does weight cycling lead to more rapid weight gain and predispose one to binge eat? Or, does binge eating simply increase as adiposity increases?

Hyperresponsivity to food palatability is greatest during the kind of moderate restriction found in most weight loss regimens. This hyperesponsivity leads to overeating, which contributes to the development or maintenance of obesity (Wooley, Wooley & Dyrenforth, 1979). Furthermore, Stunkard's (1974) review of fasting and calorie-restricted diets has found that moderate intake is more difficult to tolerate than a total fast.

Elevated free fatty acid levels are characteristic of sera of the obese (Bjorntorp, Bergman & Vanauskas, 1969). Hibscher and Herman (1977) have found such elevations to correlate with restraint in both obese and normal weight individuals, indicating that perhaps it is disordered food intake that causes the elevation, not obesity itself. Rossner and Bjorvell (1987) followed 98 obese subjects before weight reduction, at six months, and at one year. Mean weight reduced from 120, to 105, and then to 100 kg over the one-year period. The effect of weight reduction on serum cholesterol was mixed. At six months, subjects had significant reductions in total cholesterol, VLDL, LDL and HDL cholesterol. The latter drop was undesirable. At one year, VLDL remained below pretreatment levels but LDL and HDL cholesterol were higher than at pretreatment.

The metabolic adaptations have been discussed earlier in the "Weight Regulation" section. These adaptations implicate dieting as a cause of weight gain. Brownell et al. (1986) have compared rats maintained as obese on a high-fat diet with obese rats who cycled through two periods of restriction and refeeding. During the second restriction phase, weight loss occurred at half the rate and regain at three times the rate of the first cycle. At the end of the experiment, the cycled animals had a fourfold increase in food efficiency compared with non-cycled obese rats. This suggests that frequent dieting makes subsequent weight loss and maintenance more difficult—that dieting contributes to weight gain and obesity.

There is some evidence in the literature that even when weight loss is achieved in the obese, there is no improvement in body image disturbance, self-esteem, or the perception of self in terms of fatness (Glucksman & Hirsch, 1969; Stunkard & Burt, 1967; Stunkard & Mendelson, 1967). Thus, not only does weight loss through dieting fail to improve some of the psychological realities of obesity, but it may worsen the physical ones. In addition to the physical and emotional effects of dieting listed above, repeated failure at attempted weight loss can only serve to reaffirm low self-worth and self-esteem. In conclusion, there is evidence to support the notion that not all obese women should be repeatedly dieting to attempt weight loss. It seems not only ethical to suggest weight maintenance as a goal, but perhaps unethical to continue to advise repeated dieting.

ALTERNATIVE INTERVENTIONS TO DIETING

If continued dieting is not advisable, what are the alternatives for the obese? As indicated in an earlier section of this review, there have been few trials attempting to change body dissatisfaction, and none of these have been directed toward obese women. Therefore, the literature was reviewed in relation to the development of an intervention that would allow an alternative to dieting for obese women.

The full program content is detailed in Chapter 3, and literature related to the description and purpose is outlined below. Two interventions were developed. One consisted of a large-group education session that lasted one hour per week for 12 weeks. The content presented the controversies of the literature as previously reviewed: definitions of obesity, its multiple etiologies, regulation of weight, set-point, health risks, cultural desirability for thinness, failure of different treatment methods, negative consequences of dieting, and factors affecting self-esteem and body dissatisfaction. In addition, the concept of restrained eating and strategies to normalize eating as described by Polivy and Herman (1983) were included.

From a cost-effectiveness perspective, it was felt that large-group sessions would be more economical if the educational intervention proved to be as effective as a more intensive intervention strategy.

The more intensive intervention was conducted in a small group over a two-hour period every week for 12 weeks. The same educational content was delivered, but sessions also included assertiveness training, practice at changing faulty cognitions, body image exercises, and the development of a supportive group environment.

Using Rosenberg's (1981) concept of self-esteem, an intervention was developed to improve the social interaction of the obese with significant others. In providing a group leader, credibility was established by having an expert with whom to check out perceptions of the self. The group leader became a new expert, a credible source of accepting, positive attitudes toward the obese. The development of support in the group allowed for each group member to become a "significant other" for others' self-concept, thereby positively influencing self-esteem (Meisenhelder, 1985).

Further, one component was directed at decreasing body dissatisfaction and increasing self-esteem by enhancing the physical presentation of self. A "Queen-size" model who served as a positive role model, conducted a class on the optimal use of makeup and of styles and color in wardrobe selection. Support for this intervention came from Cash's work on the relationship between the use of cosmetics and self-esteem: use of cosmetics indicated a certain minimum level of self-worth and regular use worked to enhance self-esteem even more (Cash & Cash, 1982).

Another role model, a clinically obese, but very fit, female fitness instructor conducted one session about the emotional and physical benefits of fitness (Folkins & Sime, 1981). Thereafter, participants were asked to report the activity they had done during the week and were encouraged to commit themselves verbally to mild exercise before the following session.

Assertiveness training was added to the more intensive group in order to allow practice in responding to inevitable bias and discrimination against obesity. In a small before-after study, participants had rated their bodies as more active and stronger after assertiveness training (Cottraux, Mollard & Defayolle, 1982).

The use of cognitive therapy in treating body image dissatisfaction has been described and tested in a randomized trial by Butters and Cash (1987). It was found to be effective, with maintenance of effect at seven-week follow-up. Therefore, cognitive methods were incorporated in this intervention to help women correct negative assumptions and beliefs such as "I am fat. Therefore, I do not have a right to be happy in life."

Interventions were directed to decreasing the centrality of body shape and appearance in determining self-esteem. These included: identifying ways in which the body functions well for the person, and allows for functional, social, and pleasurable aspects of life; identifying aspects of self that are highly positive and making those a focus (for example, a good mother, wife, worker, friend); determining that weight loss would not "change my life"—financial status, roles, skills would not be any different after a 50-pound weight loss. Thus, the program was directed to normalizing eating, increasing self-esteem, and decreasing body dissatisfaction and the importance of body size in determining self-worth.

3

Beyond Dieting:
The Weekly Program

INTRODUCTION

This chapter has been developed so that a health professional could take the outline provided here and actually conduct the "Beyond Dieting" intervention. Included are specific exercises, content areas covered each week, and discussion of participants' reactions to the process at specific times in the program. The content areas are indicated without including all details of the content as they are found in the literature review (Chapter 1). Handouts that have been used are included as appropriate. Suggestions are given for other materials that have been found to be helpful.

The non-dieting approach described here is a psychoeducational group. As such, this chapter is merely a suggested outline and is not meant to be adopted rigidly. The "first-time" leader will find it useful to follow this outline, but gradually, with practice and familiarity with the content and exercises, the leader will devise the program that suits his or her own style and meets the needs of each individual group. Each group will have its own pace and will bring forward content at different times. For the most part, the group leader should use principles of adult education and go in the direction the group participants seem to need at the time. Occasionally, the group needs some background information in order to deal with a question that has been raised currently. In that case, the leader must explain that other background information is needed that will evolve over the next few weeks, and that the group will definitely get an answer to the question over the course of the following few weeks. This situation tends to happen more frequently in the early stages of the program when the need of the group is to know everything at once.

Cognitive therapy techniques are useful in this group. They have been explained to participants, or the group leader may simply model the questioning of underlying assumptions, giving other possible explanations and self-talk in response to a negative, derogatory self-statement. As in any group, people come to the group with different needs. Occasionally, it becomes evident that a participant has needs for therapy that are beyond the scope of the program. The group leader should discuss with that individual, in private, options for other therapy: either concurrent or before continuing in the group. Concurrent therapy with the group leader is not recommended because of potential changes in the group dynamics. Therefore, the group leader must have sources of referral where the therapists are in agreement with the philosophy of the program objectives.

Some participants may inquire about individual therapy at completion of the group. Again, options can be explored with them. It may be enough to offer an ongoing support group for monthly meetings after completion of the 12 weeks. In the experience of the Beyond Dieting program, the support group is an option that about 10% of participants took. In addition, with permission of all involved, the names and contact information for each group member is distributed early in the 12 weeks. This allows for ongoing contact on a less formal basis. Some participants have developed their own support group that meets for dinners and socializing.

As a general rule, it is helpful to watch the media and to ask group members to bring in newspaper and magazine articles, books and tapes, or accounts of television or radio programs that support both dieting and non-dieting. This sharing of current news and views will help participants to develop their own ability to critically analyze claims for the latest fads.

The ideal group size seems to be about eight people. Therefore, it is realistic to start with 10 to 12 participants to allow for drop-outs. Larger groups do not allow for individual discussion of issues and of problems related to eating and accepting body shape. Smaller groups are lacking in a range of experiences, consequently there is less chance for participants to identify with someone else's experience of the same things—to feel that they are not the only ones who have felt a certain way. Group membership is kept closed throughout the 12 weeks for group consistency.

The program as described here has been used only with women to date, although about five percent of phone calls of inquiry in response to the media advertising were from men. At the end of every 12-week session, the participants were polled on the issue of having a group of men and women combined. The overwhelming majority felt the program should continue to be conducted with same-sex groups only. The author would be happy to hear from anyone who conducts the program with men or with mixed groups.

Another issue that has not been evaluated is the actual body shape of the group leader. Beyond Dieting was evaluated with all groups conducted by the author, who is of very average size and has never had a weight problem. After the evaluation component, other leaders were trained, partially through attendance at a 12-week session with the author. New group leaders have been mostly past "graduates" of Beyond Dieting (therefore, obese) who have education and clinical experience in a health profession such as social work or psychology.

From the perspective of group leaders, it has been ideal to have the combination of the average-size author and "graduate" coleaders. We need to formally evaluate the differences in effect of leaders of different size. The large-size graduates hold the power of a role-model for participants. However, some participants initially are skeptical of this, attributing less credibility to content of the program and seeing the content as a rationalization on the part of the leader. Further, they anticipate that the leader will "brainwash" them with the same rationalizations.

ADVERTISING AND PUBLICITY

Participants were solicited by advertisement, "lifestyle" news articles in the three local newspapers, and guest appearances on local television and radio talk shows. The newspaper articles were, by far, the most effective means of generating interest in the program. The author simply called the newspaper and asked to speak to an editor so that contact could be made with the appropriate writer. Departments to which the author was referred varied at each newspaper among "lifestyle," "health," and "women's issues." Writers were very cooperative in writing articles about the program—it seemed to be a topical, interesting area to them.

The writers usually asked to come to the group to observe, meet, interview, and photograph the participants. The writers remained cooperative even when these requests were denied. It was explained that this was a very sensitive area for the individuals involved, and that inclusion of a one-time only observer/reporter might inhibit the group or therapeutic process. Group members often did not initially want friends and relatives to know that they were attending this group. Therefore, they certainly did not want pictures taken. Several group members did agree, in the latter part of the 12 weeks, or after completion of the entire program, to be interviewed as to the process they had experienced in the group.

As a trial, a 2″ by 4″ advertisement was purchased and appeared two consecutive Saturdays in the "life-style" section of one newspaper. This ad generated about eight phone calls. By contrast, one no-cost interview that covered about half of the front page of a midweek "life-style" section generated 400 calls. Television and radio appearances resulted in anywhere from five to 100 calls each, depending on the popularity of the station. Cooperation of the media was essential to the success of this program.

As the study progressed, word spread among the various health care providers in the city. Family physicians and various therapists started to refer clients to the program. These referrals were not accepted into the evaluation component of the study, but were invited to join subsequent groups. The referred participants often seemed to be more "needy" than the self-referred clients.

INFORMATION SESSION

Potential participants are always invited to attend an information session prior to committing themselves to a 12-week program. It is a large commitment for most people, and there is an effort to maintain the group membership by ensuring that they are very aware of the purpose and goals of Beyond Dieting before signing up. The one-hour session reviewed the following areas:

1. This is *not* a diet program.
2. The purposes of the group are to reestablish normal eating, improve self-esteem, and learn to deal with our own and others' negative messages about our body shape in order to be more accepting of ourselves.
3. The program is specifically for "overweight" women who have been chronic dieters in the past, but who have not been successful in maintaining weight loss. It may be necessary to discourage those who are of quite average weight or even thinner than average. It is not an appropriate group for them, as the heavier attendees will look upon them with the attitude of "What are you doing here?" They may, in fact, get quite a hostile reception. Those people who came to the group but were judged not to be eligible were given information about a "body image" group in the local area which was dealing with some of the same issues around acceptance of body shape and weight. It was felt to be more effective to keep the group more homogeneous, to register only those women in the higher weight range. A height/weight table was developed that gave ranges of weight 120-200% of average based on a national table of average weights by age and sex. The table was used as a reference guide in making the decision about registering or referring women to the other body image group.

4. The process of the group:
   - small group format, two hours/week for 12 weeks;
   - expectation of learning new content and new ways of responding to various situations;
   - expectation of participation in discussion, time for individual questions and progress reports;
   - combination of information sharing, discussion, group, and individual exercises about body image, self-esteem;
   - cost (estimated to recover hourly fee to group leader, may need to cover rent, advertising if necessary).
5. The major content areas of the 12 weeks:
   - cultural/media pressures to be thin, resulting prejudice;
   - effects of dieting on mood, behavior, eating patterns;
   - set-point evidence, and metabolic adaptations to dieting;
   - normal eating—what it is and how to achieve it;
   - self-improvement—exercise, make-up, clothing;
   - evidence regarding health risks of obesity;
   - body image, self-esteem.
6. Body size of group leader: Explain the advantages and disadvantages of having different-size leaders and be open to questions.
   - large-size leader—advantage is that she acts as a positive role model for the participants, as someone who has struggled with dieting and weight issues and is now accepting of herself and size; disadvantage is that participants may see the content as the leader's rationalization for lack of success in weight loss and maintenance;
   - average-size leader—advantage is that content is not seen as a rationalization, contributes to credibility of the content; disadvantage is that leader cannot entirely relate to the extent of struggles with dieting and prejudice experienced by the group participants. However, the point can be made that few women in our society have escaped dieting or body dislike at some point in their lives, and the shared experiences can come from the group.

It should be made clear to information session attendees that if they feel they cannot live with the body-size implications of the group leader, they should not join.

WEEK 1

Objectives

At the end of Week 1, the participants will be able to:

1. feel comfortable in the group, and know at least the first names of three people;
2. describe the group norms;
3. describe the purpose of the 12-week program, and at least five areas of content to be covered;
4. explain how "ideal" body shape for women is culturally determined.

Group Process Issues

1. Introduce group leader, her qualifications and related experience (can again raise issue of own body size, struggles with body image and weight).
2. Introduction of group members: What about the advertising attracted their attention? What made them decide to participate?
3. Group norms—expectation that participants will attend each week or let group leader know that they are not coming.
   - Get agreement that all information shared will be confidential and will not be discussed outside of the group.
   - Participants will ask questions when they are not clear about any information given; no question is a "dumb" question.
   - If they are asked to give responses to a particular question or exercise, it is very acceptable to "pass" if they feel uncomfortable with sharing the information at that time.

4. Initiate a discussion and decision about word to be used in the group to describe size—possibilities include "obese," "fat," "overweight," "queen-size," "larger," etc. Explain that the word will not be used in a pejorative sense but simply as a descriptor of body size.

Group Exercise—Dreams and Nightmares

Ask participants to anonymously write down three topics they would like to have discussed over the next 12 weeks (their dreams of the ideal class), and their goals in attending. Also have them write down what topics they hope will be avoided during the 12 weeks (their nightmares), i.e., "I'm so tired of reading and hearing about . . ."

The group leader will review the papers and acknowledge which topics will be included and discussed in the program, i.e., review the topics to be addressed, with rationale for inclusion/exclusion of topics which participants have indicated are undesirable/desirable.

Usual reactions of participants:

1. Dreams
   • to be able to give up bingeing;
   • to learn to live with myself, not put life on hold until I lose weight;
   • to be able to eat something in front of others without feeling guilty;
   • to lose weight.

2. Nightmares
   • to have to hear about another diet or food guidelines such as nutrients in each food;
   • to have to count calories again;
   • to have to write down everything we eat;
   • will gain weight.
   (Note: the leader will have to remind participants that this is *not* a weight loss group.)

Content—Cultural Imperative for Thinness in Women

The group leader will lead a discussion about the effect of culture of the "diet-obsessed" society on women; the current pressure to be thin and ideas for how that evolved, history of "ideal" body shapes for women, variation today of the ideal shape from one culture to the next, glamorization of eating disorders, and prejudice against obese. Include the fact that the basis of prejudice in our society is based on the false assumption that all obese people can do something about their weight, but are choosing not to do so.

Questions that promote discussion include: What is the media stereotype about thin women, fat women? Have you been in contact with other cultural groups where being large is valued? What have been your experiences of discrimination as a large woman—in employment, travel, eating, shopping for clothing?

Homework

1. Be aware of stereotyping of large and thin women in the media and report back next week.
2. Report any instances of discrimination you have experienced over the week.

Leader Resources

1. This book, Chapter 1, sections "Cultural drive for thinness" and "Stigmatization of the obese."
2. Garner, D. M., Rockert, W., Olmsted, M. M., et al. (1985). Psychoeducational principles in the treatment of bulimia and anorexia nervosa. In D. M. Garner & P. E. Garfinkel (Eds.), *Handbook of Psychotherapy for Anorexia Nervosa and Bulimia*. New York: Guilford Publications (pp. 515–523).
3. Polivy, J., & Herman, C. P. (1983). *Breaking the Diet Habit*. New York: Basic Books, (pp. 12–26).

WEEK 2

Objectives

At the end of Week 2, participants will be able to:

1. describe their own decision-making related to starting, continuing, or stopping a diet, and relate relevant factors that go into each decision;
2. understand the effects of dieting on eating, mood, behavior, physical symptoms, and anthropometric measurements;
3. relate the effectiveness of reducing diets.

Review of Previous Week

Discuss examples participants bring regarding media stereotypes of fat and thin women.

Hear and discuss examples of discrimination experienced over past week. How was it responded to by the group member? Are there any suggestions for other responses that might have been effective? (Note: this is a good time to introduce the idea of assertiveness and how it differs from passive acceptance of discrimination versus hostile or aggressive responses. Indicate that more time will be spent on assertiveness in a later session.)

Group Process Issues

The end of Week 2 is often a good time to ask whether participants are willing to have their names, addresses, and phone numbers distributed to the group, so that individuals may call each other regarding issues between classes and build in support for each other. Include the work number of the group leader as another reminder of how you may be contacted if members are not able to attend one week. Pass sheet of paper for willing participants to write address and telephone numbers, then photocopy list for distribution the following week.

Group Exercise—The High Cost of Dieting

Participants will take a moment with paper and pencil to add up how much money they estimate that they have spent on dieting in the past year, the past five years, their lifetime. Include formal programs, diet supplements, food replacements, drugs, diet books and magazines. Share these figures among the group and try to get a total amount of money for the group over the past year, five years, and lifetime. The point should be made that the diet industry is a huge, profitable business that has little long-term effect for most individuals, beyond profit-making for others.

Group Exercise—The Decision to Start/Stop a Diet.

Discuss decision-making related to dieting. The purpose is to raise awareness and share experiences. Everyone has the right to choose to go on a reducing diet. What events or feelings occur that lead to the decision to attempt to reduce? (Examples might include admonishments from family to lose weight, or a shopping experience when it was difficult to find attractive clothes that fit properly.) Questions to promote discussion include:

How do you feel, physically and emotionally, at the beginning of a diet? Do you feel an initial sense of power and control over your body? How long does that feeling usually last? How do you feel when you reach a plateau and you do not lose any more weight even though you still restrict your intake? Do you feel any physical or emotional changes after a period of time on the diet?

Content—Effects of Dieting

The group leader will promote discussion to bring out the following effects of dieting.

1. On eating: heightened external cue responsiveness, hyper-responsivity to food palatability (greatest during periods of mod-

erate restriction, more hunger on moderate restriction than total fast, period of restriction leads to bingeing).

2. On mood: fatigue, irritability, depression, hysteria and hypochondriasis, nervousness, outbursts of anger.

3. On behavior: social withdrawal, reduction in libido, increase in other "oral" behaviors (nail-biting, smoking, gum-chewing), impairment of concentration, alertness and comprehension.

4. On physical symptoms and anthropometric measures: gastrointestinal discomfort, dizziness, hypersensitivity to noise, light and cold, decreased strength, decreased metabolic rate, temperature, pulse and respiratory rate, loss of body weight, fat and muscle mass (however, on refeeding, weight and fat return but muscle mass does not return without exercise).

5. On weight loss (effectiveness of reducing diets): 60–95% of attendees at outpatient weight loss treatment regain weight lost within one year, many have rebound increase in weight by that time due to metabolic depression during calorie restriction.

Discussion questions:

What was the longest time you were able to keep at reduced weight following a loss? Have you known many people who were able to lose significant amounts of weight and maintain that weight loss? Many of the above points can be raised by asking participants to relate their own experiences with reducing diets.

Resources

1. This book, Chapter 1, sections "Attempted treatments of obesity and outcomes" and "Effects of dieting."

2. Garner, D. M., Rockert, W., Olmsted, M. M., et al. (1985). Psychoeducational principles in the treatment of bulimia and anorexia nervosa. In D. M. Garner & P. E. Garfinkel (Eds.), *Handbook of Psychotherapy for Anorexia Nervosa and Bulimia*. New York: Guilford Publications (pp. 523–532).

3. Polivy, J., & Herman, C.P. (1983). *Breaking the Diet Habit.* New York: Basic Books, (pp. 75–99, 129–157).

WEEK 3

Objectives

At the end of Week 3, the participants will be able to:

1. understand the theory of set-point;
2. be aware of the metabolic adaptations the body makes in reaction to attempts to change weight from one's own "natural" weight;
3. be aware of their own emotional reaction of ambivalence to this information—feeling relief and frustration with the thought that dieting may not work for them.

Review of Previous Week

1. Ask if there are any questions about the effects of dieting.
2. Hand out phone list.

Content—Set-Point Evidence

Focus of this session will be on presenting information about set-point. Discuss early studies of Keys et al. (1950) and Sims et al. (1973); make participants aware of metabolic reduction that occurs as an adaptation to calorie restriction, rebound weight gain after dieting, evolutionary sense of set-point allowing survival of our ancestors in periods of food scarcity.

Usual Reactions of Participants

The information about set-point and metabolic adaptations to calorie restriction is usually new to most participants. The reaction is initially one of relief—they feel that their bodies have somehow known this all along, but now they know it "intellectually" as well. There is relief in realizing that another reducing diet is not the answer, that they do not have to force themselves through another period of deprivation and discomfort from not eating.

Many group members go quickly (i.e., during the same session) from relief to wanting to know, "Then how can I lose weight?" "If dieting does not work, what is the answer?" There currently is no good way to lose weight and keep it off. The ideal, in the absence of an effective weight loss program, is to change one's goal from weight loss to *health,* to normalizing eating and improving self-esteem, to get on with life instead of putting life on hold until 40 pounds are lost. It is important to reassure the group that set-point implies that weight will not continue to increase forever, but will level off with normal eating. One encouraging likelihood is that group members are above set-point as a result of long-term dieting with its metabolic depression. Therefore, a period of normal eating may result in some weight loss (10–20 pounds). Regular physical activity may also slightly reduce weight and tone (inches). Again, this does not mean 40 pounds will be lost. It is important not to set up unrealistic expectations at this point, but also, to not leave members feeling that this is a hopeless situation. This group tends to be quite inactive, so it should be emphasized that activity does not mean a strenuous, painful program, but means simply movement such as dancing to music in the privacy of their bedrooms, or walking for 15 or 20 minutes, three to four times per week.

Tell members that the focus for the next week is on defining and returning to normal eating.

Resources

1. This book, Chapter 1, sections on "Weight regulation," and "Attempted treatments of obesity and outcomes."
2. Garner, D. M., Rockert., Olmstead, M. M., et al. (1985). Psychoeducational principles in the treatment of bulimia and

anorexia nervosa. In D. M. Garner & P. E. Garfinkel (Eds.), *Handbook of Psychotherapy for Anorexia Nervosa and Bulimia.* New York: Guilford Publications (pp. 532–541).

3. Polivy, J., & Herman, C. P. (1983). *Breaking the Diet Habit.* New York: Basic Books, (pp. 27–53).

WEEK 4

Objectives

At the end of Week 4, participants will be able to:

1. understand the overall process of return to "normal eating";
2. identify where they are in the process and set goals for achieving the next step;
3. understand the value of "normal eating" in reducing binge eating and increasing the quality of food intake.

Definition.

For the purposes of this program, "normal eating" is defined as the eating of three meals a day, with snacks between meals if meals are more than 3–4 hours apart. It includes eating a variety of foods of high quality (following national dietary recommendations of high unrefined carbohydrates, low fat, high fiber), as well as occasionally eating foods that would have been "forbidden" on a reducing diet" such as pastries and "junk food" and eating these foods without guilt or danger of disinhibition and subsequent overeating of such foods. It also includes eating food of sufficient quantity as to be emotionally and physically satisfying.

Review of Previous Week

Discuss variations in emotional reactions to information about set-point in order to bring out vacillations and ambivalence between the "good news" (I do not have to go through that deprivation again because the chances are slight that it will be permanent weight loss), and the "bad news" (but I do not want to stay at this weight forever).

Content—"Normal" Eating

As a result of long-term dieting, participants usually come to the Beyond Dieting program with one of two eating patterns. One is that they believe that they will weigh less if they eat one meal a day. Invariably, because of the social function that meals play, this one meal is the evening meal. The problem is that once they start eating it is very difficult to stop. So they eat their meal and continue snacking until bedtime, consuming the same number of calories (and often of lower quality) as they would have if they had eaten meals and snacks throughout the day.

The other pattern is to go on a calorie-restricted diet each Monday. The restriction lasts until Thursday or Friday (long enough to begin the metabolic reduction), then they overeat all weekend to compensate for the physical and emotional deprivation of the week. By the time Monday comes again, their guilt about overeating is such that they are even more stringent with restriction at the beginning of the week, which leads to greater disinhibition of restraint the following weekend. Both patterns are likely to result in maintenance of a higher weight than eating a more regular pattern of three meals a day and a few snacks.

In the group, it is helpful to talk about these two patterns of eating to get some idea of how typical they are of the participants. Help them to realize that, as a result of this pattern of restraint and disinhibition, their weights could be higher than if they ate regularly. A regular pattern of intake keeps regular periods of diet-induced thermogenesis and thus keeps their metabolic rate more stable.

Participants will be presented with strategies to normalize eating. The author's clinical observation is that the most effective way to achieve "normal eating" is by following, in order, the steps presented below. That is, ensure that one phase is established and comfortable before going on to the next. Assure participants that people take different times to achieve each step, that each week there will be time for individual discussion regarding where they are in the process, with ongoing assistance. Some may reach the end of the 12-week session still working on the first phase, but they will be well aware of strategies to get through the next phases of "normal eating."

a) Give up dieting

Eat three meals per day, initially, to retrain the recognition of hunger and satiety. The regular pattern seems to induce conditioning of the physiological signals of hunger to occur at mealtimes. If meals are more than three hours apart, a fruit or juice snack between meals is helpful to keep from arriving at the next meal famished—which often leads to rapid eating with ingestion of more food than would otherwise be eaten. Ask participants not to be too concerned at this point with the quality or quantity of the food eaten, but to focus on establishing the pattern. Tune in to your body and allow yourself to recognize hunger. Respond by eating a meal or nutritious snack.

b) "Forbidden" foods

There is no such thing as a "forbidden food" as those lists appear on diet sheets. Eat a variety of all foods in moderation. In order to be able to eat previously forbidden foods such as cake or ice cream, without overeating, it is helpful to eat these items only after a meal. That is, one is more likely to eat several servings of a dessert if one attempts to eat a serving *instead* of a meal. Direct the participants to deal with guilt by stating to themselves that this is normal eating, this will allow them to eat regularly without bingeing on "forbidden" foods after a period of restriction. This is a cognitive therapy example of challenging their underlying belief that because they are fat, they should not eat at all, let alone eat desserts.

c) Overall food intake

When (a) and (b) are comfortably established, participants can begin to focus more on the quality and quantity aspects of their food intake. Group members have usually shown in-depth knowledge of what they "should" be eating. That is, they have a sound knowledge base of good nutrition. However, here, as with any exercise, they demonstrate dichotomous thinking. They are either *on* a diet or *off* a diet. When *on*, they are very restrictive, eating only vegetables and fruit, low-fat meats, few bread and cereals and no sweets. *Off* a diet, they eat little meat, fruits or vegetables, much junk food and sweets. The goal here is to combine these two eating patterns, eating moderately from all types of foods.

A brief review of good nutrition usually suffices. Pamphlets may be procured from a dietitian or from a nutrition division of the local hospital or health department. References may be given for nutrition books for the general public for those who want more information.

Quantities of food should be eaten to leave the individual feeling satisfied—neither "stuffed" nor still hungry. In order to learn this, participants should be encouraged to experiment with different sizes of servings. Try smaller portions, and ask oneself if that was "enough." They should be able to respond that they could still fit more food into their stomachs, but that they are no longer hungry. It is important that they acknowledge the emotional satisfaction of food, to eat food that they enjoy. It will require some self-talk to be able to stop eating before the stomach is uncomfortably full. When they are eating previously forbidden foods, participants should be asked to remind themselves that this is *not* the last time they will eat this food item (as is often the message before starting on a diet), but that more can be obtained tomorrow, if desired then. It may also help to cook smaller portions during this experiment, to avoid the compulsion to "clean up"—to not leave leftovers or throw out food.

Some behavioral techniques learned in dieting to slow down eating are useful in learning to recognize satiety. These include putting down the fork between each mouthful, eating only in one place, and eating with full concentration on food instead of watching television or reading at the same time. Again, frequent self-talk is involved, for each woman must ask herself if she is comfortable yet with the amount of food taken—neither still hungry nor too full.

Resources

1. This book, Chapter 1, section on "Effects of dieting" regarding restrained eating.
2. Polivy, J., & Herman, C. P. (1983) *Breaking the Diet Habit.* New York: Basic Books, (pp. 190–211).

WEEK 5

Objectives

At the end of Week 5, participants will be able to:

1. realize that they are worthy of the time and energy investment in order to feel more comfortable with their appearance.

Content—Self-Improvement

The social pressures to be thin in today's society impose an ideal on overweight women, an ideal that is unrealistic for many. Yet, the media give constant messages about new diet and exercise regimens that promise weight loss at last! So, women embark on yet another attempt at weight loss and are disappointed to find that, once again, it has not resulted in permanent weight loss. Thus, many fat women have learned from their repeated failure to dissociate from their bodies which have caused them such humiliation and rejection. This alienation and low self-esteem may result in a lack of motivation to take responsible care of one's physical life and health. It may even inhibit active participation in social and work life.

Why should a fat woman take care of her body if it has such a negative value to her? Her thinking may be that if she cannot be slim, and therefore, healthy and beautiful, there is no point in making any effort in the directions of health and self-presentation.

In order to counteract some of this thinking, this program will include information about self-development and self-improvement in the areas of makeup, the use of different colors and shapes of clothing to enhance appearance, and exercise. Self-improvement will be presented not as a trivial feminine pursuit, but as serious interventions to improve self-esteem and fight against discrimination.

Explain the above reasoning for inclusion of this workshop, and introduce the guest resource person.

Usual Reactions of Participants

Group members are often initially reserved as they find the resource person a bit intimidating at first. Most have not spent time learning correct application of makeup or considering their own personal style in clothing. The reservation gives way eventually to active experimentation in the workshop.

Resources

Find a female resource person in your area who is able to present a "workshop" format in two hours about the use of makeup and of clothing color and styles to enhance image. It is preferable to get someone who is, herself, larger than average, if not obese. This will present a powerful role-model for the participants. A source of such a person is usually a large-size modelling agency. Large-size models value their appearance and size and, therefore, are good candidates for a resource for this session, if they are comfortable presenting in front of a group.

Buying suitable clothing is often an issue for large women— finding shops that sell clothing that fits, in a price range that they can afford. The market has been improving over the past few years, but it is helpful to have a sharing time during this session to discuss area stores for shopping.

"Large-size" specialty shops may be another source for the resource person for this session. They may hold the workshop at their store after hours, and actually allow group members to try on various colors and styles of clothing. This has worked well for Beyond Dieting if it is clearly negotiated with the manager beforehand that this will be an "experiment" for the participants, and they will not be expected to buy clothes during the workshop session. If interested, group members may return at a later date to make purchases. This relieves the pressure for sales, and the pressure to buy on the part of the participants.

Resources

1. Roberts, N. (1985). *Breaking All the Rules*. New York: Penguin.
2. Magazines—"Big, Bold & Beautiful" ("BBB"), and "Radiance," two U.S. publications that beautifully present large women. (Note: It is helpful to have a few issues available, particularly of BBB. Member reactions are often surprised by the fact that large models are used and that they can agree that the models are attractive. This is another challenge to a long-held belief of theirs that large size equates with unattractiveness.)

WEEK 6

Objectives

By the end of Week 6, participants will be able to:

1. identify where they are in relation to the process of normalizing eating, and set goals for achieving the next step;

2. understand the concepts of body image and self-esteem, and how they are related;
3. understand that they may be able to see their bodies more neutrally, less negatively, at some point in the future.

Review of Previous Week

1. Ask for feedback regarding last week's session, particularly about resource person.
2. Spend about 30 minutes asking members about their experiences during the week in achieving goals set for return to normal eating. Allow group to give suggestions and support to each other, problem-solving together about related issues. Have each person state what her goal is for the next week to bring her closer to normal eating.

Content—Body Image and Self-Esteem

Components of self-esteem will be presented. Body image will be presented as one component of self-esteem. Obese women have a tendency to discount positive aspects of themselves because they are obese.

Encourage members to give up tape measures and scales. Many people allow the step on the scales each morning to dictate how their day is going to go. If below the magic number, the woman goes through the day with confidence and a positive outlook, but if above the magic number, the woman is self-berating, self-denying, and gloomy for the day.

Questions that promote discussion:

Name some women from politics, the media, movies who are large women and are positive role models. How does size affect their performance in their job? What is body image? What does it mean to over or underestimate body image? How stable is it? How does it relate to overall self-esteem? What are other components of self-esteem in addition to body image? What do you think of when you think of the word FAT? THIN? (Use cognitive therapy strategies to change participants' underlying assumptions to more neutral or positive ones.)

Group Exercise—Body Image

1. White paper that comes in rolls and is about three feet wide can be cut into six-foot lengths and taped to the wall. Have participants stand facing the paper, mark the top of their heads on the paper, then stand back and draw life-size silhouettes of themselves.
2. Have another participant superimpose actual dimensions by tracing each woman's body on her piece of paper. Then each participant is left with her first guess regarding her own body shape along with the actual body outline on the same paper for comparison.
3. Discuss in the group how the two markings differ for each person. It is expected that some will underestimate their body size, but most will overestimate. What do these differences mean to each participant?
4. This exercise is particularly helpful for women who overestimate their body size. The point can be made that they can change their self-talk when thinking that they are too large to re-membering that this exercise has demonstrated that they are not as large as they see themselves.

Group Exercise—Getting Life Off "Hold" and Going

The purpose of this exercise is for participants to realize that they may be in the habit of putting off goals or responsibilities in life until the day that they are the ideal body shape.

1. Ask members to write on a piece of paper all of the things that they are waiting to get thin before they do (examples

include wearing a belt, eating an ice cream cone in public, buying clothes, visiting long-time friends, joining an exercise class, returning to school, leaving or entering a relationship).

2. Participants publicly commit themselves to doing one thing over the next week, that they would normally not do unless they were thinner. Repeat this exercise the next week with a riskier activity. Encourage participants to behave as though they are comfortable with their bodies.

Homework—Body Awareness Exercise

Obese women tend to avoid looking in the mirror, or they look only at their face and do not look at the rest of their body. Have the participants, at home, use a means to relax them—soft music, warm bath, time to lie quietly on the bed, or progressive muscle relaxation (Benson, 1975). When relaxed, they should look at their body in underwear, or nude, if they are able. Just observe the body for neutral observations such as skin color in various parts of the body, patterns of hair distribution, how far down their legs their fingers touch, etc. When they notice their attention going to judgments of body parts, such as "my thighs are too big," redirect sight and thoughts to neutral thoughts. Try this exercise at least once, preferably three times over the next week. This is simply a body awareness exercise to reacquaint the participant with her body. Note: Many participants will not have a full length mirror. They may do this exercise in a changing room of a clothing store if they are able to take time to relax before beginning.

Resources

1. This book, Chapter 1, sections on "Self-esteem," "Body image," and "Relationship of satisfaction with appearance to self-esteem."
2. Benson, H. (1975). *The Relaxation Response.* New York: William Morrow.

3. Hutchinson, M. G. (1985). *Transforming Body Image.* New York: Crossing Press.
4. Sanford, L. T. & Donovan, M. E. (1985). *Women and Self-Esteem.* New York: Penguin.

WEEK 7

Objectives

At the end of Week 7, the participants will be able to:

1. identify where they are in relation to the process of normalizing eating and set goals for achieving the next step;
2. realize the controversy in the literature regarding the health risks of obesity—that they are not necessarily at greater risk of dying because they are overweight.

Review of Previous Week and Homework

1. Get feedback from the group regarding any further reactions to the body drawing exercise.
2. Report back to the group about the homework of doing some activity as though they were comfortable with their bodies, something they would previously only have done if thinner.
3. Report back regarding homework of looking in the mirror and practicing neutral observations. (Note: Some participants may not have been able to bring themselves to do this because they are so uncomfortable with the idea of looking at themselves. Ask them to try again this week, fully clothed, and gradually over the weeks to reduce the amount of clothing. Reassure them that there will be some other exercises in the program that may help them do this exercise at a later date.)
4. Review again where each participant is in the process of normalizing eating and involve group in problem-solving for the difficulties each woman is facing.

Content—Is Obesity a Health Risk?

The purpose of this session is to present the controversies in the literature about the health risks of obesity. It is usually a more didactic session as the participants will not have the information to share.

Massive obesity (over 100% above ideal weight) is definitely a health risk. (Reassure participants that they would not have been eligible for this group if they fit this category).

However, debate is evident in the literature as to the extent of risk involved in being less than 100% above ideal weight. Is obesity an independent risk factor or merely an associated factor to other risk factors? Does obesity cause poor health or just statistically happen together with some diseases?

Simopoulos and Van Itallie (1984) concluded that overweight persons die sooner than average weight persons and that obesity is an independent predictor of cardiovascular disease. However, Brunzell (1984) argues that a significant portion of the risk of obesity on coronary artery disease is mediated through specific familial disorders that are associated with both obesity and premature coronary artery disease. Andres (1980) reviewed the major population studies of obesity and mortality and found that they failed to show that overall obesity leads to any greater mortality risk. He even suggests that moderate obesity may be associated with some benefits.

The Framingham study (Hubert, Feinleib, McNamara & Castelli, 1983) found that conditions such as emphysema and suicide are less frequent in the overweight group than in those underweight. There is some evidence that heart disease, diabetes, and hypertension may be due to weight fluctuations, and are thus more common in the overweight who continually attempt to reduce their weight, rather than being due to the obesity alone. In addition, family history (heredity) is a more critical risk factor in determining morbidity and mortality than weight.

More recent research has focused on distribution of body fat. It indicates that health risks are greater if fat is distributed in the abdominal area than if fat is in the hip and thigh area. The location of fat distribution is more important than the amount of fat in determining health risk. If the waist measurement is greater than hip measurement, the risk of morbidity and mortality is increased.

Resources

1. This book, Chapter 1, section on "Obesity as a health risk."
2. Polivy, J. & Herman, C. P. (1983). *Breaking the Diet Habit.* New York: Basic Books, (pp. 54–74).
3. An annotated bibliography (Appendix E) may be given out to participants to give to their family physicians if their physicians are pressuring them to lose weight despite lack of identified medical problems.

WEEK 8

Objectives

At the end of Week 8, participants will be able to:

1. describe the benefits of physical activity;
2. verbalize a concrete plan for what physical activity they will do for periods of 10 minutes, three times over the next week.

Review of Previous Week

1. Discuss any questions or reactions regarding the information of the health risks of obesity from last week.
2. Review specific questions only in relation to normal eating, as the time for this session should be primarily allotted to the physical activity content and experiential practice.

Content—Physical Activity

This session will focus on the benefits of physical activity. Fat people can be fit! The role of exercise in weight reduction will be deemphasized, focusing attention on movement as pleasurable activity.

Time should be taken to discuss the myths that all average weight, or thin people are fit, and that all obese people are unfit. Also, the group leader or resource person should deal with the dichotomous thinking that is characteristic of this group of women who believe that if they cannot run six miles, or do an advanced level of aerobics class, then anything less is worthless and they do no physical activity. Exercise benefits include:

1. mood enhancement, stress reduction, reduction in depression— the effect is more pronounced in subjects who are more distressed or physically unfit at the outset of beginning an exercise program (De Vries, 1968; Folkins, Lynch & Gardner, 1972; Morgan, Roberts, Brand & Feinerman, 1970).

2. self-concept improvement (shown in 3 randomized controlled trials) (Hilyer & Mitchell, 1979; Martinek, Cheffers, & Zaichowsky, 1978; McGowan, Jarman & Pederson, 1974).

Group Exercise

The resource person will lead the discussion about the benefits of exercise, types of classes and exercises to avoid, and how to begin a moderate activity program. She will acknowledge that most obese women have not exercised on a regular basis and usually prefer not to go to a class because of difficulty "keeping up."

About 45 minutes will be spent on a very low-intensity exercise session. This will include demonstration of exercises to do and to avoid. It will be primarily stretching, moderate strengthening, and a very mild aerobic session, keeping in mind that the aerobic capacity of the women will likely be limited. Participants should be monitoring their heartbeat.

Several different approaches have been taken to prepare the group members for this session. Generally, our experience has been that if the group is told the week before that there will be a mild activity component to Week 8, some participants choose not to attend. Most have a long history of aversion to exercise. The most successful approach has been to not tell participants about the session in advance. Therefore, they come in their usual street clothing, without proper shoes. The resource person needs to know that this is the case in order to plan an appropriate session. This means that most activities are done on the spot, without jumping or quick movement. At the end of the session, each member will commit to doing some activity for 10 minutes, three times over the next week. Emphasize that activity should be easy to fit into schedule, not require other people, equipment, or club membership, and one that participants will find at least neutral, if not enjoyable.

Resources

The local recreation centers, YMCA, YWCA, high school physical education departments, or fitness clubs can usually direct the group leader to a female fitness instructor who is larger than the stereotype. The larger fitness instructor can be a powerful role model, reinforcing the message that fat can be fit!

WEEK 9

Objectives

At the end of Week 9, participants will be able to:

1. identify where they are in relation to the process of normalizing eating and set goals for achieving the next step;
2. identify reasons they eat, or have eaten in the past, other than hunger, and some alternative strategies to eating under those circumstances;
3. realize that there are many causes of obesity besides overeating or underexercising;
4. acknowledge that there is no characteristic "obese personality."

Review of Previous Week

1. Review individual's activity for the past week. Discuss barriers or problems experienced, using group input to deal with same. Discuss activity goals for each person over the coming week.
2. Review individual's progress toward "normal eating." The group leader might be able to incorporate in this discussion the content, below, on eating when not hungry.

Content

Eating when not hungry.

Ask individuals to recount times of awareness of eating when not hungry. Do they eat because of stress, procrastination, boredom, loneliness, frustration, anxiety, or happiness and celebration? One strategy is to stop the automatic eating in relation to a feeling of emotional discomfort. Eating may have become automatic as it provides some short-term relief, distraction, or pleasure. The strategy involves taking time out before reaching for food, between meals, to ask if one is truly hungry. If the answer is yes, the next strategy is to define what one really would like to eat at that time.

Often, group members report wanting something that would have previously been forbidden, such as a chocolate. If that is what one really wants at the time, it is best to satisfy that urge. What often happens is that they often double-think themselves into eating celery instead, find they still are not satisfied so they eat fruit, and are still not satisfied so they eat a muffin. In the end, they have eaten more calories in bypassing what they really wanted than if they had eaten some chocolate in the first place.

If the answer to the question about hunger is that they are not hungry, then one needs to take some quiet time to think about what it is they really want. Is it that they need a way to relieve their stress, anxiety, or boredom? Brainstorm with the group alternatives to deal with each emotion or situation, especially alternative ways to reward themselves. Food in our society is often used as a comfort or reward. Take time to figure out what is pleasurable for the body; stop denying pleasure through stringent dieting.

Causes of obesity and the myth of the "obese personality."

What causes obesity? Is there an obese personality? The literature is full of conflicting information.

Sclafani (1984) reviewed the animal literature and found 50 distinct known causes of obesity involving neural, endocrine, pharmacologic, nutritional, environmental, seasonal, genetic, viral, and ideopathic mechanisms. Many of these mechanisms may be present in humans.

Similarly, obesity has been related to personality disorders and dysfunctional families (Bruch, 1973; Kaplan & Kaplan, 1957). However, in a recent review, McReynolds (1982) concluded that these relationships have been a function of the particular population studied. "Obese persons who are unselected with respect to physical health and psychiatric status function as well as or better than comparable nonobese persons. Research does not support a psychology of obesity based on psychoneurotic or psychosomatic process."

Schacter (1971) hypothesized that obese people were "externally controlled," that they responded to cues in their environment that led them to eat, rather than to "internal" body cues. Herman and Polivy (1975, 1980, 1984) further researched this hypothesis, but found that the difference was not "internal-external" but rather that of "restrained-unrestrained." People who weighed more were often more "restrained" in their eating patterns, but then became "disinhibited" and overate.

Homework

Practice stopping self from automatic eating long enough to ask if hungry. If not hungry for food, identify emotional state and consider alternatives to eating at that time.

Resources

1. This book, Chapter 1, section on "Obesity—Definition, measurement and etiology."
2. Polivy, J. & Herman, C. P. (1983). *Breaking the Diet Habit.* New York: Basic Books, (pp. 129–155).
3. Roth, G. (1984). *Breaking Free From Compulsive Eating.* New York: Signet.

WEEK 10

Objectives

At the end of Week 10, participants will be able to:

1. identify where they are in relation to the process of normalizing eating and set goals for achieving the next step;
2. name at least five things they can appreciate about their body;
3. give assertive responses (as opposed to passive or aggressive responses) to practice scenarios regarding weight and dieting issues.

Review of Previous Week/Homework

1. Review specific questions only in relation to normal eating.
2. Review progress of stopping automatic eating and finding alternative actions in relation to specific emotional states or situations.
3. Ask if there are any questions related to last session's content regarding the myth of the "obese personality" or regarding causes of obesity.

Content—Self-Esteem and Body Appreciation

The content of this session should come out of the exercises listed below. They are designed to illustrate the issues of body appreciation and self-esteem, and assertiveness.

Group Exercise—Self-esteem and body appreciation

1. It took years to develop current feelings about their body. Therefore, it will take time to develop a more positive attitude. Ask participants to brainstorm regarding things that their bodies currently do very well for them. The group leader may need to start the group off with examples of functioning in physiological, locomotor, or interpersonal areas (groups often fail to appreciate even sexuality or reproduction).

2. Next have each woman make a list of personal accomplishments that have been unrelated to weight. Share at least one of these per person with the group. The purpose of this exercise is to develop a positive list of functions and attitudes related to oneself, to enhance self-acceptance and self-esteem from accomplishments unrelated to body shape.

3. The last phase of this exercise is to engage the group in the discussion of what would be different in their lives if they were 40 or even 100 pounds lighter. Would their jobs or relationships with coworkers, children, or family be improved? The advertising for weight loss programs perpetuates the myth that weight loss will change the world for the individual. In reality, little beyond clothing size would change for most women.

Group Exercise—Assertiveness

Ask the group to give examples of common experiences related to their weight (e.g., salespeople telling them they could not possibly fit into any of the clothing in their store, family members telling them, "You should not be eating that"). You cannot do anything about a past incident but you can be prepared for the next. Discuss alternative ways to handle similar incidents in the future.

Resources

1. Roth, G. (1984). *Breaking Free From Compulsive Eating*. New York: Signet.

2. Hutchinson, M. G. (1985). *Transforming Body Image*. New York: Crossing Press.

WEEK 11

Objectives

At the end of Week 11, participants will be able to:

1. identify where they are in relation to the process of normalizing eating and set goals for achieving the next step;
2. recognize that they are experiencing loss and are grieving the loss of the dream to be thin.

Review of Previous Week

1. Review specific questions or problems with the process of normalizing eating.
2. Review body and self-appreciation. Discuss with members any instances over the past week when they found themselves thinking about things they or their bodies do well.
3. Review with group any examples that came up in the past week when they had a chance to practice assertiveness skills.

Group Exercise—Decision-Making Regarding Return to Dieting

Divide a blackboard, overhead, or flip chart into two columns. Label one "Advantages of continuing dieting" and the other "Advantages of following a non-dieting approach such as Beyond Dieting." Get group to brainstorm advantages and disadvantages of each. Discuss ownership—that the decision is theirs. With different pressures at different times, the decision will have to be remade a number of times.

Content—Loss

One of the disadvantages of the Beyond Dieting approach is that it means the loss of the dream to be thin. This involves a grieving and adjustment process.

Discuss the concept of loss. Ask participants what they have to lose by giving up severe dieting? What will they lose if they like their bodies? Will some relationships be threatened, such as a diet partner or family member? Will they have to give up the illusion that all would be well in life, love, and work if they just weighed 30 lbs. less?

Ask participants to relate other experiences of loss and what strategies helped them to cope and adapt. Strategies such as exercise, time out (vacation), distraction, and support of others usually emerge from this discussion. Focus some discussion of the importance of social support. Who is supportive in their lives now? What is support? How do you recognize when you need it? How can you go about getting it? When, and what kind of help is helpful? Acknowledge that members of this group are a very strong source of support in relation to body and food issues. Encourage them to use their phone lists and to call, or arrange visits with each other to keep up the support that they experience in the group.

Homework

Ask group to come prepared the following week to ask questions for clarification or about gaps they are experiencing as this will be the last opportunity in the group. Reassure the group that there can be phone contact with the leader for questions, if you are willing. Also relay information about an ongoing support group if you will offer one.

WEEK 12

Objectives

At the end of Week 12, participants will be able to:

1. identify where they are in relation to the process of normalizing eating and set goals for achieving the next step;
2. feel that they have had a chance to clarify any ambiguous issues or content.

Review of Previous Week

1. This session should include an in-depth review of where each individual is in normalizing eating. Group input to problem-solving is essential.
2. Discuss issue of loss again. Suggest that the group set a time to get together socially for ongoing support.

Content—Summary Session

The group leader will review the educational issues from previous weeks and review "dreams and nightmares" exercise from the first week to see how the program did or did not address the issues desired by the women. Suitable references will be given for those subjects not addressed. Questions will be received from the group for review or new explanations as they feel necessary.

A process evaluation of program will be done. An example is given in Appendix D.

4

Evaluation of the Program

PURPOSE

As stated in the introduction, the primary purpose of this project was to develop an intervention that would allow obese women to deemphasize the importance of body size in determining self-worth, thereby increasing self-esteem and decreasing the restrained eating patterns that accompanied ongoing attempts to reduce their body size.

A randomized trial was initiated to evaluate the intervention. In light of cost considerations, two such interventions were developed. Both groups met once per week for 12 weeks. The "Education" group consisted of a large-group format (16-21 women) that was delivered in lecture style and included only the educational content. The group labeled "Experiential" was more a more intensive psychoeducational group. It consisted of a small-group format (6-8 women), met for two hours per week, and included the educational material, cognitive therapy strategies, assertiveness, and body image exercises, as well as a group support component. Details of the interventions are in Chapter 3: Intervention.

The evaluation was made up of several measures of physical, psychological, and social health. Three hypotheses were tested.

HYPOTHESES

1. Participation of obese women in a group "Education" intervention program

    a) increases self-esteem

    b) decreases body dissatisfaction

    c) decreases restrained patterns of eating.

2. Participation of obese women in a group "Experiential" intervention program

    a) increases self-esteem

    b) decreases body dissatisfaction

    c) decreases restrained patterns of eating.

3. Participation in the "Experiential" intervention will result in

    a) increased self-esteem

    b) decreased body dissatisfaction

    c) decreased restrained patterns of eating

    which are of greater magnitude than results of participation in the "Education" intervention.

4. Any post-intervention changes that occur in self-esteem, restraint, or body dissatisfaction from either intervention will be maintained at six-month follow-up.

Secondary Outcomes of Interest

Much controversy and emotion surrounds the issue of fat as presented in Chapter 1: Background Literature. It was decided that several secondary outcomes should be examined in this study to investigate whether a non-dieting approach does more harm than good. Therefore, all participants were followed for scores on depression, bulimia, drive for thinness, and social adjustment scales. Physiological measures were also taken to see if weight, blood pressure, glucose, and lipids would be altered, as compared to a control group.

SUBJECTS

Participants were solicited by advertisement, "lifestyle" news articles in the three local newspapers, and guest appearances on local television and radio "talk" shows. As the study progressed, word spread among various health care providers in the city. Family physician and psychiatrist referrals started to appear. The decision was made to not include these referrals until the study was complete, for the sake of maintaining as much homogeneity as possible. That is, it was expected that participants who came as a result of referral would likely be different in psychological profile from those who were self-referred.

The investigator met with the volunteers prior to the beginning of the program to explain the purpose of the program and to ensure that the following criteria were met. Participants were female, over 20 years of age, at 120-200% of ideal weight (Health and Welfare Tables), able to obtain their doctor's consent, and willing to come to the program for two hours once per week for 12 weeks. Volunteers excluded were those who were pregnant, as pregnancy is a time of rapid body change. Women were also excluded who had a medical or psychiatric disorder self-disclosed or known to their family physician. The intent was to have a healthy population.

A letter concerning the nature of the program was sent to the volunteer's physician to gain consent in writing for the patient's participation in the program and to verify that the exclusion criteria did not apply. Explanatory letters ensuring confidentiality of all information were provided to the participant and her physician. Signed informed consent was obtained from each participant and her physician.

Following signing of the consent form, the participants completed the pretest questionnaires, had their weight, height, and blood pressure measured, and arranged with their family physicians to have a blood sample taken for fasting glucose and lipids. The same questionnaires and physical assessment measures used in the pretest were used as posttest measures immediately following the 12th session, at six and 12 months. The wait-list control group completed posttests at 12 weeks, then attended the subsequent session without waiting for the six-month time period.

Calculation of sample size for statistical significance suggested that at least 30 women were required to complete the program in each of the three groups. The drop-out rate was projected to resemble that of most weight loss programs (20-50%). Therefore, an intake of about 150 volunteers was targeted (to allow for a 40% drop-out).

A table of random digits was used to randomize participants to one of three groups: the "Education Group," the "Experiential Group," and the "Control Group." Participants who had been randomized to the control group were delayed in starting the program by 12 weeks and were telephoned for the posttest and start of the next program.

INTERVENTION

Details about the actual process and content of the intervention are contained in Chapter 3 of this book. A brief outline will be given here for the purposes of understanding the evaluation. The program began in July, 1986, under the auspices of the National Eating Disorder Information Centre (NEDIC) in Canada. Initially, the groups were held in a meeting room at the community-based location of NEDIC, then they moved with NEDIC to Toronto General Hospital (March, 1987).

The "Education Group" was delivered one hour per week for 12 weeks to a total of four groups of 18-21 women. It provided information on weight regulation and its implications for dieting, the lack of evidence that obesity is a significant health risk on its own, the cultural imperatives regarding body shape for women, and the effects of dieting on emotions and eating style. Food issues focused on strategies to return eating to a non-dieting state. In addition, the relationship of body shape to self-esteem was outlined.

The "Experiential Group," a psychoeducational group, had this package plus other interventions such as body image exercises, cognitive therapy exercises, group support-building, and assertiveness. This group was delivered two hours per week for 12 weeks to a total of seven groups of 6-8 women.

Estimates of time spent on each topic were recorded at the end of each of the 12 sessions for both interventions to allow comparison of time per topic across the interventions. Process evaluations (Appendix D) were completed by participants at the end of the final session of the intervention.

INSTRUMENTATION

A number of instruments were chosen to assess social, behavioral, and attitudinal dimensions of body shape and self-esteem, any of which could have been affected by participation in the intervention. Economy, ease of administration and scoring, and objectivity of scoring formed the basis for selecting self-report measures. However, there are cautions to be considered with any self-report scales. Inaccurate reporting (through misinterpretation or deliberate over or under representation) and response-set bias may occur.

The following questionnaires were administered:

1. Self-esteem measures:
   • Janis and Field's Feelings of Inadequacy Scale
   • Rosenberg Self-Esteem Measure (RSE)
2. Eating and weight-related measures:
   • Three-Factor Eating Questionnaire (TFEQ)
   • Restraint Scale
   • Eating Disorder Inventory (EDI)
3. Depression
   • Center for Epidemiologic Studies—Depression Scale (CES-D)
4. Social adjustment
   • Social Adjustment Scale—Self-Report (SAS)

The entire package took, on average, 40 minutes to complete. The ordering of scales in the package of questionnaires was altered to prevent fatigue for particular questionnaires.

Many self-esteem measures exist. A global measure was sought for this study, and the Janis and Field and Rosenberg scales were chosen as they have had more testing in terms of reliability and convergent and discriminant validity than the Coopersmith or Tennessee scales (Wylie, 1979).

Diet diaries of daily intake were considered as a direct means of assessing if the amount and pattern of intake changed as a result of the intervention. However, a major anticipated outcome was that the participants would become less obsessed with food and thoughts of eating. Therefore, a diet diary was considered counterproductive, and more indirect measures of eating behavior were sought. The Restraint Scale (Herman & Polivy, 1980) and the Three-Factor Eating Questionnaire (Stunkard & Messick, 1985) both are reported to identify dieting behavior.

Janis and Field—Feelings of Inadequacy Scale

This 20-item scale is a measure of global self-esteem in the sense of feelings of social adequacy (Janis & Field, 1959). Convergent validity has been demonstrated through correlations with other self-esteem measures. The version used in this study was revised by Eagly (1967). Internal reliability has been demonstrated to be high with a split-half reliability estimate of 0.72, Spearman-Brown reliability of the total test was 0.84. The possible score range is 20–100.

Rosenberg Self-Esteem Measure (RSE)

The RSE is a global measure of self-esteem, with special reference to the evaluation the individual makes and maintains about himself or herself regarding an attitude of approval or disapproval (Rosenberg, 1965, p.5). Consisting of 10 items, each rated on a four-point scale ranging from strongly agree to strongly disagree (possible scores range from 10 to 40), it is a quick test to administer and score. In addition, it has high reliability (two-week test-retest reliability coefficient = 0.85) and demonstrated convergent validity with three different self-esteem measures (correlation coefficients from r=0.56 to 0.83) (Wylie, 1979).

Restraint Scale

Herman & Mack (1975) developed this scale as a way to identify dieters in their early studies of externality. Revised by Herman & Polivy (1975), the 10 items assess the degree to which one purposefully tries to restrict food intake for weight control or weight reduction. The Restraint scale contains items to assess both weight fluctuations and subjective concern for dieting.

There are some problems in using the Restraint Scale with the obese. As many as 90% of obese are restrained (Herman & Polivy, 1980) when the usual cutoff score of 16 is used as in the general college female sample. Significant correlations of restraint and percentage overweight have been found when using the Restraint Scale with obese populations (Lowe, 1984; Ruderman, 1983), but it is not clear if the higher score is due to greater weight fluctuation or if it reflects frequent, intermittent dieting (Heatherton, Herman, Polivy, King, & McCrea, 1988). There is also reduced reliability for the obese. For example, when investigating internal consistency, Ruderman (1983) has found coefficient alphas of 0.86 for normal weight and 0.51 for obese subjects.

However, the questionnaire has the power to predict consistent group differences in dieters and nondieters in terms of their restrained eating patterns and the subsequent disinhibition which follows from restraint (Heatherton, Herman, Polivy, King, & McCree, 1988). Because the Restraint Scale has been useful in studying behavior that characterizes dieters, irrespective of weight loss (Heatherton, et al., 1988), it was used as a potential indicator of change in dieting behavior in this obese sample.

Three-Factor Eating Questionnaire (TFEQ)

This factorially-derived questionnaire was developed through combination, factor analysis, refinement, and further testing of the Restraint Scale (Herman & Mack, 1975) and a similar tool, the "Latent Obesity" scale (Pudel, 1975). Stunkard and Messick (1985) found three factors of eating behavior: cognitive restraint, disinhibition, and susceptibility to hunger. Test-retest reliabilities for the factors ranged from 0.80 to 0.93. The same authors found that the scales all discriminated between dieters versus free eaters beyond the 0.001 level, except for the disinhibition scale. However, for this scale there has not yet been a behavioral validation of restrained eating style in producing counterregulation, as has been demonstrated for the Restraint Scale.

When the TFEQ was compared with the Restraint Scale, there was a significant correlation between the "cognitive restraint" and the "tendency to disinhibition" scales which did not occur with the "perception of hunger" scale (Heatherton, 1986). Heatherton et al. (1988) have concluded that the TFEQ may measure successful restraint or successful dieters, while the Restraint Scale may measure all who are attempting to restrict their food intake. That is, the Restraint Scale measures people who restrict their intake for a time, then are disinhibited (at least temporarily freed from their restraint) and subsequently overeat. The same authors hypothesize that the TFEQ identifies styles of eating rather than identifying dieters; "restraint" in TFEQ is indicative of a degree of food restriction, rather than a range of behavior exhibited by most dieters as measured by the Restraint Scale. Thus, it was decided that for this study both scales would be used as they seemed to measure different aspects of eating behavior and cognitions.

Eating Disorder Inventory (EDI)

This self-report scale was designed to assess behavioral and attitudinal characteristics clinically observed in anorexia nervosa and bulimia (Garner, Olmsted & Polivy, 1983). Its 64 items are divided into eight subscales: drive for thinness, bulimia, sense of ineffectiveness, perfectionism, interpersonal distrust, interoceptive awareness, maturity fears, and, of most interest in this study of obese women, body dissatisfaction. Reliability (internal consistency) and convergent and discriminant validity have been established for all subscales. In earlier studies, an obese group had significantly higher "body dissatisfaction" scores than an anorexic, formerly obese group or a control group. The obese group also had significantly higher scores than the control group on the "bulimia" and "drive for thinness" subscales (Garner, Olmsted & Polivy, 1983).

Center for Epidemiologic Studies—Depression Scale (CES-D)

This self-report "state" measure of depressive symptoms (Radloff, 1977) consists of 20 items concerning four primary factors: depressed affect, positive affect, somatic symptoms, and interpersonal symptoms. It was developed for use in epidemiologic surveys of depression within the general population, and thus was chosen over the Beck Depression Inventory (Beck, Ward, Mendelson, Mock & Erbaugh, 1961), another commonly used depression scale, as the Beck was developed for, and has been used largely in clinical populations. The CES-D is not a diagnostic instrument; it provides an index of cognitive, affective, and behavioral depressive features and indicates the frequency of symptoms. Internal consistency has been established; Cronbach's alphas for the CES-D total range from 0.84 to 0.90 and have now been validated in several different clinical populations and community samples (Devins & Orme, 1985).

Social Adjustment Scale—Self Report

This self-report questionnaire measures, by its 42 items, either instrumental or expressive role performance over the past two weeks in six major areas: work as a worker, housewife or student; social and leisure activities; relationships with the extended family; marital role as a spouse; parental role; and membership in the family unit. High internal consistency (0.74) and high retest reliability (0.80) have been demonstrated. Concurrent validity has been established, as well as sensitivity to change following interventions (Weissman, Prusoff, Thompson, Harding & Meyers, 1978).

ANALYSES*

As stated in the hypotheses, the major outcome variables were body dissatisfaction, and two measures each of self-esteem and restraint. Analysis of variance was used to determine if there were significant differences among the three groups at pretest on any of the measures. Multivariate analysis of variance with pretest scores as a covariate (MANCOVA) was performed, using Pillai's Trace test, to determine overall effect of each intervention group compared to the control group and to each other.

The hypotheses also indicated that the intervention groups would be followed to determine if any effects are enhanced, diluted, or unchanged six months and one year following completion of the program. A MANOVA was done with six-month follow-up data, comparing the two intervention groups only, as the control group had, at this point, been entered into an intervention. In addition, analysis of variance was done for each outcome variable by group over the first three measurement times. Fewer than half of the participants were available at one year follow-up, limiting meaningful analyses. Therefore, their mean scores and standard deviations are simply reported for the five major outcome variables.

Secondary outcome variables of interest included social adjustment, depression, two subscales of the EDI (bulimia and drive for thinness), and physical measures (weight, blood pressure, and serum levels of glucose, lipids, and cholesterol). As above, analysis of variance was done to determine if groups differed at pretest. Univariate analysis examined significant differences within and between groups at posttest and at six-month follow-up.

Regression analysis was performed to determine if there were variables that were predictive of positive outcome from the intervention, beyond group assignment. Therefore, the scores on the Rosenberg and Janis and Field scales, the two measures of restrained eating (Restraint Scale and TFEQ), and the body dissatisfaction scale

---

*All analyses were performed using SPSS/PC+ version 2.0.

of the EDI, along with pretest weight and percent average weight, were entered in a stepwise manner after group and regressed on the sum of the change in scores on the five major outcome scales from pre- to posttest time.

Pretest and posttest scores of the women who attended the six-month follow-up were compared with scores of those who did not attend. Analysis of variance was used to detect differences on the self-esteem, restraint, and body dissatisfaction scales.

Pearson product-moment correlations were calculated for body dissatisfaction and the two measures of self-esteem, for the entire sample at pretest, for the two intervention groups at posttest and at six-month follow-up. This statistic was completed to test the assumption that, initially, body dissatisfaction was central to self-esteem in this sample of women, and that body dissatisfaction could be reduced in its importance to the overall self-esteem as result of the intervention.

ATTENDANCE

A total of 17 information sessions were held. Five hundred forty-eight (548) women called the NEDIC and indicated a willingness to participate in the information sessions by giving name and phone number. One hundred seventy-eight women (178) actually attended (32.5% of those who originally indicated a wish to participate).

One hundred forty-two (142) women who attended the information session agreed to be study participants (79% of those attending). Twenty women (14% of those attending) were eligible but did not wish to join the study, and 17 women were excluded for the following reasons:

Below weight criteria	12	(7% of those attending)
Above weight criteria	2	
Had gastric stapling	2	
Unable to obtain M.D. permission	1	

Randomization resulted in the following group assignment:

	N	%
Educational	47	33.1
Experiential	49	34.5
Control	46	32.4
Total	142	100

A total of four large-group Educational and seven small-group Experiential sessions were held. After the 12-week waiting period and posttests, subjects in the control group were allowed to choose the time of attendance. They were not informed of the different structure of groups.

Posttests were administered to those subjects who attended 10 or more of the 12 sessions in the two intervention groups, and to those controls who agreed. Nineteen controls (41%) decided not to participate in the study following the 12-week wait period. Most had joined other programs, expressing their readiness to do "something" about their body or attitude toward it. At that time, "Beyond Dieting" was the only non-dieting program in the area, so the other programs were directed to weight-loss or else dealt with compulsive eating, like Overeaters Anonymous.

The pre- to posttest dropout rates were lower than expected in the two intervention groups; however, drop-out rates did achieve the expected rate of 40% at the six-month follow-up. Rates are displayed in Table I.

TABLE I

Drop-out Rates

Group	Pretest, N	Posttest, N	Drop-outs N	Drop-outs %	Drop-outs at 6 Months N	Drop-outs at 6 Months % Pretested
Educational	47	36	11	23	24	51
Experiential	49	42	7	14	29	59
Control	46	27	19	41	—	—

Descriptive Data

The descriptive information obtained on pretest is found in Table II.

As can be seen in Table II, participants were a mean age of 40 and at 148% of Canadian average weight for age, height, and sex. It is interesting to note that, as a group, participants were close to their highest weight ever, supporting their subjectively reported feeling that it was "time to do something" about their weight.

The ideal weight chosen by the subjects seemed to be influenced by their current weight in the sense that they selected a weight that was still heavy by normative standards. In this way, participants appeared to be quite realistic about ideal weight.

TABLE II

Pretest Descriptive Data

	Mean	Std Dev	Range
Age (years)	39.4	11.2	20–67
Height (inches)	65	2.7	58–73
Weight (lbs)	208.7	33.2	158–300
(kg)	94.9	15.1	72–136
Percent average weight	148%	22.7	118–200%
Lowest weight (lbs)	145	26.5	96–289
At current height (kg)	65.9	12.1	44–131
Highest weight (lbs)	217	40.0	146–332
At current height (kg)	98.6	18.2	66–151
Ideal weight (lbs)	143	15.2	110–200
(Subject perception of) (kg)	65	6.9	50–91
Age weight problem began	16	11.8	0–56

51.4% reported weight problem by age 12
62.6% by age 16
69.2% by age 20
Thirty-seven (26%) were currently on a diet.

The age of onset for obesity indicated that the majority of participants would be classified as juvenile onset, with 70% reporting a weight problem by age 20.

Nine percent of participants did not complete questions about marital status (Table III). Through conversations during the intervention phase, it became obvious that most women in the unreported category were married. Similarly, the question of husband's occupation was often not completed. Therefore, occupational status was coded based on subject's occupation alone. Occupational status was coded according to Hollingshead's scale (Hollingshead & Redlich, 1958). Seventy-four percent of participants were in categories 2, 3, or 4, indicating a predominantly middle-class status, based on their own occupation. One participant was Black, the remainder were Caucasian.

BETWEEN-GROUP COMPARISONS

Comparisons at Prettest

Analysis of variance revealed no significant group differences on any of the five major variables at entry into the program. On the variables of secondary interest, there were three significant differences at pretest. For two of the EDI subscales, bulimia and drive for thinness, the Education group had a significantly lower mean score than the control and Experiential groups ($p=0.04$ and $p=0.035$

TABLE III

Marital Status

	N	%
Married	58	40.9
Single	47	33.1
Separated/divorced/widowed	24	16.8
Unreported	13	9.2
Total	142	100

respectively, Appendices B.11 and B.12). On social adjustment, the control group had significantly poorer mean adjustment than either intervention group (p=0.0069, Appendix B.9).

Pre- to Posttest Comparisons

Analysis of variance failed to show significant differences in the control group from pre- to posttest times. Therefore, any general public education or social changes happening at the time were not powerful enough to effect a change. Any change noted in the intervention groups can thus be attributed to participation in the intervention.

Table IV illustrates the findings of the multivariate analysis for the five major outcome variables, using scores at pretest as covariates of posttest scores. Pillai's Trace statistic was used as the multivariate criterion as it is considered to be the most stringent and robust test of all the possibilities in the SPSSPC+ program (Norusis, 1988). The number of participants in each group for whom all 10 scores (five measures repeated) were available, and were thus available for multivariate analysis were: Education (n=26), Experiential (n=29) and Control group (n=23).

These analyses demonstrate that the Education group did not differ significantly from the control group when the five outcome variables were combined. However, the univariate analysis showed significant differences on the Restraint Scale and approached significance on the two self-esteem scales.

The more intense Experiential group did have significantly different overall F test results when compared with the Education and the Control groups. This indicates that the Experiential group had a greater influence in producing positive change than the Education group. The univariate analyses showed consistently improved scores in the Experiential group over the control group on both measures of self-esteem, both measures of restrained eating and body dissatisfaction. The Experiential group also proved to be significantly more powerful than the Education group on every measure except for

TABLE IV

MANCOVA—Pre- to Posttest

	Education Versus Control	Experiential Versus Control	Experiential Versus Education
Overall F	1.83	12.12	4.44
p	0.12	0.001*	0.02*

Univariate F-tests with (1,70) df:

	F	p	F	p	F	p
J&F	3.66	0.06	14.77	0.001*	3.11	0.08
RSE	2.92	0.09	18.2	0.001*	5.74	0.02*
Restraint	5.64	0.02*	48.52	0.001*	8.95	0.001*
TFEQ	0.93	0.34	11.44	0.01*	5.35	0.03*
BODYDIS	2.05	0.16	5.12	0.03*	0.53	0.48

*Indicates significance at $p < 0.05$

body dissatisfaction, and with a trend to significance on the Janis-Field Scale.

Comparison of Interventions at 6-Month Follow-up

The control group was not available for follow-up at six months as subjects were entered into an intervention at the end of the 12-week period. Therefore, only the two interventions are included in the MANOVA comparing the posttest to six months posttest. Only those subjects for whom all five test scores were available were entered into the MANOVA analysis: Education (n=21), Experiential (n=25).

Table V indicates that the two intervention groups did not differ from each other at the six-month follow-up time either on the overall F, including each of the five outcome variables, or in the univariate analysis of each variable.

TABLE V

MANOVA—Six-Month Follow-up

Education ($N = 21$) versus Experiential ($N = 25$)
Overall $F = 1.49$ $p = 0.21$

Univariate F-tests with (1,70) df:

	F	p
J&F	0.10	0.75
RSE	2.93	0.09
Restraint	0.04	0.85
TFEQ	0.002	0.97
BODYDIS	2.33	0.13

Analysis of variance of pretest and posttest scores of the five major outcome variables (for the participants who had not been randomized to the control group) revealed no significant differences between the participants who were available for six-month follow-up, and those who were not available. Therefore, at pretest and at posttest, the people who became drop-outs were not significantly different from those who stayed in the program.

INDIVIDUAL OUTCOME VARIABLES

Self-Esteem

Table VI and Figure 1 illustrate the changes in the Rosenberg Self-Esteem scores over the first three measurement times. Scores at pretest on the Rosenberg Scale were 26-28, which were below the norm of 31 reported in the literature (Rosenberg, 1965; Boldrick, 1983), indicating low self-esteem. This score was comparable to the 26.4 reported for a bulimic group (Gross & Rosen, 1988). There was a significant improvement only in the Experiential group pre- to posttest. This score went to 32 at posttest and was maintained at six months, and at one year for the few people available. It is also interesting to note that at one year the few Education group participants had also reached the level of the psychoeducational group participants.

The Janis & Field "Feelings of Inadequacy" Scale mean scores are shown in Table VII, and in Figure 2. Mean scores for the

TABLE VI

Rosenberg Self-Esteem Scale

| | Assessment Time | | | | | | | | | | | |
| | Pretest | | | Posttest | | | 6 Months | | | 1 Year | | |
Measure/Group	N	M	SD	N	M	SD	N	M	SD	N	M	SD
Education	26	25.5	5.4	26	28	5.5	21	29.6	6.4	19	32.5	4.9
Experiential	29	28.1	6.8	29	32.4	5.6	25	32.7	6	17	31.7	7.0
Control	23	26.4	6.9	23	26.7	5.9	—	—	—	—	—	—

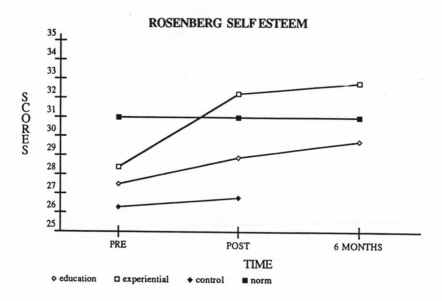

Figure 1. Rosenberg Self-Esteem Scale

control group approached those reported earlier for anorexics who were grouped by self-estimates of their body sizes into those who underestimated to moderately overestimated (mean=66) and those who were marked overestimators (mean=73) (Garfinkel & Garner, 1984). As with the Rosenberg scale, there was a significant improvement only in the Experiential group pre- to posttest. As can be seen in Figure 2, scores for the Education group continued to improve at six months whereas those of the Experiential group remained the same or may have begun to deteriorate. However, this change in the Experiential group at six months is not a statistically significantly one and does not represent a meaningful deterioration. As with the Rosenberg scale, the few available for one-year follow-up maintained their improved scores, and the Education group caught up to the same level or better.

Body Dissatisfaction

The mean pretest scores on the Body Dissatisfaction Scale of the EDI for the entire sample (mean=22) were comparable to those for an obese comparison group from an earlier study (21.1) and above anorexia nervosa patients with bulimia (17.4) (Garner, Olmsted, & Polivy, 1983). This indicates that these obese samples have greater body dissatisfaction than do patients with anorexia nervosa. Table IV illustrates that the Experiential group, but not the Education group demonstrated a significant reduction in body dissatisfaction scores as measured by the Eating Disorder Inventory. Figure 3 shows this change, and the fact that it was not maintained at the six-month follow-up. Table VIII indicates that the mean scores for those available for one-year follow-up were virtually the same as the six-month scores.

Restraint

The three scores on the Three Factor Eating Questionnaire were combined to give a total score. Again from Table IV it is clear that

TABLE VII

Janis and Field—Feelings of Inadequacy Scale

Measure/Group	Assessment Time											
	Pretest			Posttest			6 Months			1 Year		
	N	M	SD	N	M	SD	N	M	SD	N	M	SD
Education	26	62.2	13.4	26	57.4	13.6	21	51.8	14.3	19	45.5	10.3
Experiential	29	57.5	16	29	49.3	14.9	25	50.3	18.1	17	49.2	15.3
Control	23	65.2	18	23	64.4	15.1	—	—	—	—	—	—

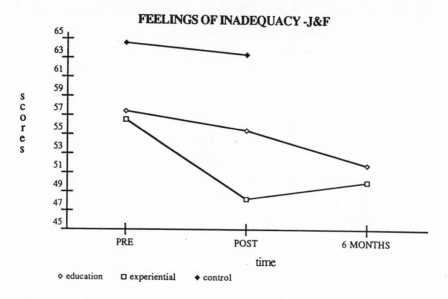

Figure 2. Janis and Field—Feelings of Inadequacy Scale

significant improvement was obtained in the Experiential group, but not the Education group on the TFEQ. By contrast, scores on the Restraint Scale showed significant improvement after both interventions. These were maintained or improved at the six-month follow-up (see Figure 4), and at one year where available (see Table IX). Initial scores on the Restraint Scale were comparable to an earlier

TABLE VIII

Body Dissatisfaction (Measured by the Eating Disorder Inventory)

Measure/Group	Pretest			Posttest			6 Months			1 Year		
	N	M	SD	N	M	SD	N	M	SD	N	M	SD
Education	26	23.5	3.9	26	19.5	6.6	21	21.3	6.4	19	22.1	5.7
Experiential	29	21.3	5.8	29	17	7	25	18.3	6.7	17	18.4	7.5
Control	23	21	5.8	23	19.3	7	—	—	—	—	—	—

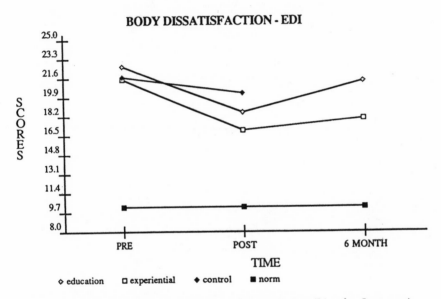

Figure 3. Body Dissatisfaction (Measured by the Eating Disorder Inventory)

anorexia nervosa sample (Garfinkel & Garner, 1984). However, scores on the Restraint Scale remained, at 18, above the score of 16 that has been suggested as the cutoff point for identifying dieters in the college population. One explanation for the posttest scores remaining high is that there is some contribution to the overall score from questions about weight fluctuation and maximum weight that could not change over the data collection time. At pretest, 95.7% of participants scored above or equal to the cutoff of 16, although, as noted in the literature review this cutoff may not be valid for the obese. (Results on the TFEQ are found in Appendices B.1-B.4)

TABLE IX

Restraint Scale

Measure/Group	Pretest			Posttest			6 Months			1 Year		
	N	M	SD	N	M	SD	N	M	SD	N	M	SD
Education	26	22.6	3.8	26	20.8	3.5	21	17.9	3.8	19	18.11	4.92
Experiential	29	23.9	3.8	29	18.3	3.4	25	18.1	5.3	17	17.65	5.58
Control	23	24	4.5	23	23	5.1	—	—	—	—	—	—

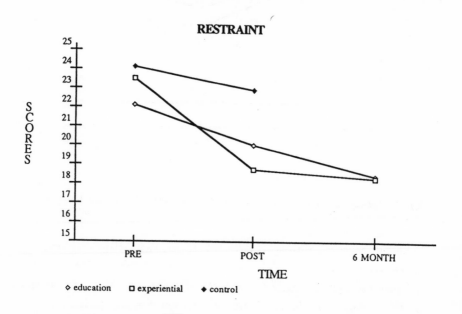

Figure 4. Restraint Scale

SECONDARY OUTCOME VARIABLES

Physiological Variables

Several physiological variables were to be assessed. The author measured weight and blood pressure at each assessment point. Also, participants were asked to have their family physician order venipuncture for fasting glucose, cholesterol, triglycerides, high density (HDL) and low density lipoproteins (LDL).

About half of the participants complied with the first request for venipuncture. However, only 27 had completed blood work at posttest, and 18 at six-month follow-up. Due to small numbers in the other two groups, only the Experiential group measurements were examined by analysis of variance. Pretest measures are found in Table X. There were no significant changes in any of the serological measures over time. ANOVA tables are found in Appendices B.5-B.8.

Blood pressure findings are reported in Tables XI and XII. There was a short-term statistically significant change in diastolic blood pressure in the Experiential group from pre- to posttest that was not maintained at follow-up.

The summary of the data on weight are shown in Table XIII, and in Figure 5. Weight and percent average weight did not change in a statistically significant way for any of the groups. However,

TABLE X

Blood Values for Experiential Group (At Pretest)

Variable	N	Mean (mmol/L)	Standard Deviation
Glucose	32	5.29	0.84
Cholesterol	29	5.69	0.99
Triglycerides	29	1.64	1.50
HDL	20	1.30	0.26
LDL	22	3.64	0.68

TABLE XI: Systolic Blood Pressure: Analysis of Variance

Measure/Group	Assessment Time									Prepost Test Comparison		Post 6 Months	
	Pretest			Posttest			6 Months						
	N	M	SD	N	M	SD	N	M	SD	F	P	F	P
Education	46	127	13.87	35	129.4	12.06	16	132.6	16.3	.3209	0.5727	0.6151	0.4365
Experiential	48	127	15.28	35	121.7	12.86	20	127.0	10.7	3.4089	0.0685	2.3660	0.1330
Control	45	124	12.73	13	127.7	11.66	—	—	—	0.8165	0.3701	—	—

TABLE XII: Diastolic Blood Pressure: Analysis of Variance

Measure/Group	Assessment Time									Prepost Test Comparison		Post 6 Months	
	Pretest			Posttest			6 Months						
	N	M	SD	N	M	SD	N	M	SD	F	P	F	P
Education	46	83	7.79	35	81	7.79	16	82.13	7.3	1.1140	0.2944	0.1419	0.7080
Experiential	48	79	7.01	35	76	6.67	20	78.6	5.6	5.0528	0.0273	1.7353	9.1934
Control	45	80	6.73	13	81	6.20	—	—	—	0.0068	0.7953	—	—

TABLE XIII: Weight in Pounds: Analysis of Variance

Measure/Group	Assessment Time												Prepost Test Comparison		Post 6 Months	
	Pretest			Posttest			6 Months			1 Year						
	N	M	SD	N	M	SD	N	M	SD	N	M	SD	F	P	F	P
Education	48	215.11	35.4	37	212.84	36.7	22	226.96	38.16	19	215	32.2	.0824	.7747	1.9839	0.1644
Experiential	49	202.39	31.8	39	205.41	34.8	26	205.15	36.34	16	201	27.1	.1802	.6723	0.0008	0.9773
Control	46	208.98	31.8	27	209.37	34.3	—	—	—	—	—	—	.0024	.9607	—	—

104

one might argue that the Education group's mean weight gain of 14 pounds from posttest to the six-month follow-up was a clinically significant weight gain. However, weight has again returned to pretest levels by one year according to those who were available for follow-up.

Social Adjustment

As previously noted, the control group had significantly higher scores (mean=2.27) on the Weissman Scale, indicating poorer adjustment than the two intervention groups at pretest. The means of all three groups were higher than the community female sample (mean=1.61) reported in the literature (Weissman, Prusoff, Thompson, Harding & Meyers, 1978). Surprisingly, the control group mean is comparable to the mean score reported for alcoholic outpatients (2.23). The two intervention groups had mean scores comparable to those reported for outpatient schizophrenics (1.99). As a total group at pretest, 89% scored above the community sample mean

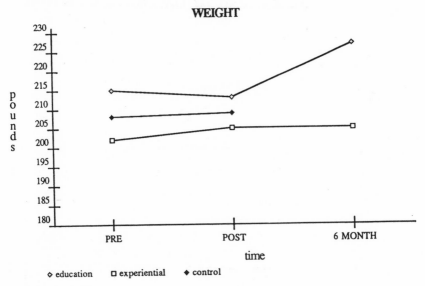

Figure 5. Weight

score of 1.61; 53% scored above the mean for schizophrenic patients; and 31% scored above the mean for alcoholic patients.

Analysis of variance (Appendix B.9) revealed a significant improvement ($F=4.608$, $p=0.035$) only in the Experiential group at posttest. This was not maintained at the follow-up. The mean score remained closer to the patient mean score than the community sample. Figure 6 illustrates overall changes in the three groups.

Depression

Pretest scores on the CES-Depression Scale were surprisingly high, indicating a high reporting of depressive symptoms. As can be seen in Figure 7, all three groups had mean scores above the suggested cutoff (16) for mild depression. The mean score for the control group was at the level suggested for moderate depression (21); however, it must be emphasized that this still does not represent the presence of depression as a syndrome. The community mean

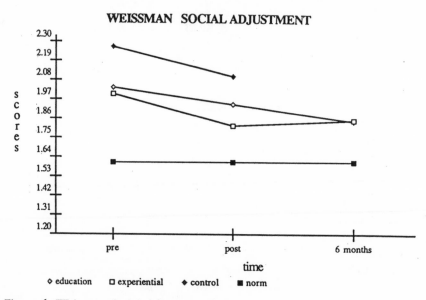

Figure 6. Weissman Social Adjustment Scale

reported in the literature is a score of 8.5 (Radloff, 1977). At pretest, 81% of all participants scored above this community mean; 60% scored above the suggested cutoff for mild depressive symptoms; 39% scored above the suggested cutoff for moderate depressive symptoms; and 15% scored above the suggested cutoff for severe depressive symptoms (31).

Analysis of variance (Appendix B.10) revealed that only the Experiential group had a significant improvement in depression scores (F=4.577, p=0.0352), but this was not maintained at six months posttreatment. However, both interventions managed to reduce scores on the scale to those equal to or below the suggested cutoff of 16.

Bulimia

The Education group had significantly lower mean scores (F=3.32, p=0.04) on the Bulimia subscale of the EDI than the other two groups at pretest. The score of the Education group was comparable

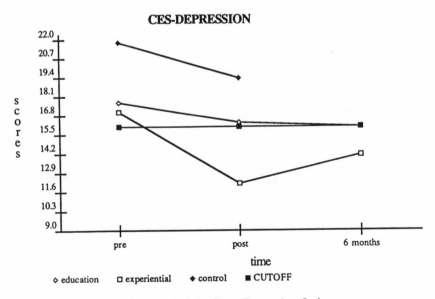

Figure 7. Center for Epidemiological Studies—Depression Scale

to the obese population (mean=4.6) and higher than female controls (mean=2.0) reported in the initial reliability and validity testing of the EDI (Garner, Olmsted & Polivy, 1983). All group mean scores were lower than means reported for the anorexia nervosa, bulimic subgroup (10.8), but higher than the restricter subgroup (2.7) (Garner, Olmsted & Polivy, 1983). Both intervention groups displayed significantly lowered bulimia scores (Education group: F=14.06, p=0.0003; Experiential group: F=58.03, p=0.0001), indicating a more normal pattern of eating. This effect was maintained at six-month follow-up, as is evident in Figure 8 and was maintained at one year for those who reported for follow-up. ANOVA tables are found in Appendix B.11.

Drive for Thinness

At pretest, as on the bulimia scale described above, the Education group's mean score was significantly lower (that is, more normal)

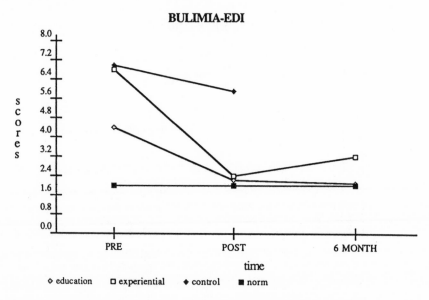

Figure 8. Bulimia Scale (Measured by the Eating Disorder Inventory)

than the other two groups. The Education group mean score was the same as the mean score for the obese comparison group described in the initial validation study of the Eating Disorder Inventory. All three groups had lower scores than the anorexia nervosa norm of 15.4 reported in the literature (Garner, Olmsted, & Polivy, 1983). Again, as for the bulimia scale, both intervention groups demonstrated significant pre- to posttest changes (Education group: $F=23.93$, $p=0.0001$, Experiential group: $F=55.89$, $p=0.0001$, Appendix B.12). There is some regression in scores at six months which continues at one-year follow-up (see Figure 9). However, the scores are still improved over pretest scores (see Appendix B.12).

REGRESSION ANALYSIS

As stated in the analysis section, regression analysis was performed to determine if there were variables that were predictive of positive outcome from the intervention, beyond group assignment. Therefore,

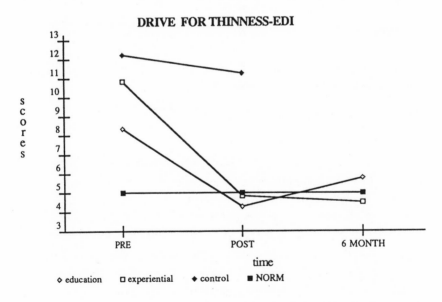

Figure 9. Drive for Thinness Scale (Measured by the Eating Disorder Inventory)

the scores on the Rosenberg and Janis and Field self-esteem scales, the two measures of restrained eating (Restraint Scale and TFEQ), and the body dissatisfaction scale of the EDI, along with initial weight and percent average weight were entered in a stepwise manner after group and regressed on the change in scores on the five major outcome scales from pre- to posttest.

The results of the regression analysis reveal that the single best predictor of total change in scores was group assignment [$F_{(2, 75)}=10.53$, $p=0.0001$], accounting for 22% of the variance. Two other significant predictors were the Janis and Field and Restraint scores at pretest. Each of these variables contributed another 9% to the shared variance, for a total (with group assignment) accounted for of 40% of the variance.

CORRELATIONS OF BODY DISSATISFACTION WITH SELF-ESTEEM

In order to explore the concept of the centrality of body dissatisfaction to self-esteem in this sample, Pearson product-moment correlations were calculated for the scores on body dissatisfaction, the Rosenberg Self-Esteem Scale, and the Janis and Field Feelings of Inadequacy Scale, using all three groups at pretest, and the two intervention groups at posttest and follow-up. As can be seen in Table XIV there were small, but statistically significant correlations at pretest between the two self-esteem measures with body dissatisfaction, indicating a direct relationship between body dissatisfaction and feelings of inadequacy (J&F) and an inverse relationship of body dissatisfaction and self-esteem (the RSE). This effect was no longer significant following the intervention, supporting the assumption that the intervention effected a reduction of importance of body satisfaction in overall self-esteem. At 6-month follow-up, there was again a significant negative correlation between body dissatisfaction and self-esteem (RSE), but no relationship with the Janis and Field scores. Appendix C shows the correlations by group over the three measurement times. With the smaller number of participants entered in the calculations, only the Experiential group had small, but significant correlations of body dissatisfaction with the Janis and Field measure at pretest. All other correlations were nonsignificant.

PROCESS EVALUATION

Two methods were employed to evaluate the intervention in a process mode. These included a time/content analysis to compare how the time was spent on each topic for each intervention. The other method involved reviewing feedback forms that were completed by each participant at the end of the last session.

Table XV compares the two interventions on total time and percent time spent on each topic. As can be seen in the table, both groups spent the most time on self enhancement and normal eating. "Self talk" was part of the cognitive therapy intervention of the Experiential group and was not included for the Education group.

TABLE XIV

Correlations of Body Dissatisfaction with Self-Esteem Measures

	Janis & Field	Rosenberg	Body Dissatisfaction
Pretest (includes all three groups)			
Janis & Field	1.0000	−0.8221**	0.3348**
Rosenberg	−0.8221**	1.0000	−0.2652*
Body dissatisfaction	0.3348**	−0.2652*	1.0000
Posttest (includes two intervention groups)			
Janis & Field	1.0000	−0.6946**	0.1497
Rosenberg	−0.6946**	1.0000	−0.2396
Body dissatisfaction	0.1497	−0.2396	1.0000
Six month (includes two intervention groups)			
Janis & Field	1.0000	−0.7867**	0.2890
Rosenberg	−0.7867**	1.0000	−0.3407*
Body dissatisfaction	0.2890	−0.3407*	1.0000

*Indicates significance at $p < 0.01$
**Indicates significance at $p < 0.001$

All other topics were comparable in the percent of total time spent on each.

Feedback received on the process evaluation forms (Appendix D) was quite positive. Every topic was consistently rated as "somewhat"to "very" "useful/interesting." Group size was rated as "too big" with "too little" time for discussion more often by the Education than by the Experiential group. With regard to the length of the program, the most frequent response for both groups was "O.K.," with other responses indicating a wish for a longer program. Rating of the group leader was consistently "good" on all three criteria of understanding of the topic, enthusiasm, and interest. Review of responses to the question: "What aspect of the program had the greatest effect on your attitudes or behavior?" indicated that information about

TABLE XV

Time/Content Analysis

Content	Education Group		Experiential Group	
	Minutes	% Total Time	Minutes	% Total Time
Introduction	10	1	20	1
Normal eating	100	12	225	16
Cultural pressure/bias	35	4	75	5
Effects of dieting	70	8	90	6
Set point/metabolism	80	10	140	10
Self-improvement	*240	29	240	17
Health risks	50	6	105	7
Etiologies	70	8	75	5
Exercise/activity	75	9	130	9
Loss/grieving	35	4	50	3
Support	20	2	60	4
Self-talk	0	0	65	5
Nutrition	25	3	110	8
Body image	30	4	55	4
Total	840	100	1440	100

*Both interventions included two two-hour sessions about use of colors, makeup, and styles to enhance self-image to others and the self.

set-point, cultural pressures, and normal eating was most important. Participants wished more time could be spent on issues such as sexuality and body image. Other suggestions for improvement included family involvement, and production of a workbook/notebook to keep track of all exercises and handouts.

SUMMARY

The results have been summarized according to the original hypotheses.

Effect of Education

The Education group did not have a significant effect on improving body dissatisfaction. It approached a significant level of improvement in self-esteem on both the Rosenberg Self-Esteem and Janis and Field Feelings of Inadequacy scales. These scores continued to improve at six months and one year post-intervention. Education did have a significant improvement on eating pattern as measured by the Restraint Scale, but not on Stunkard's Three-Factor Eating Questionnaire. The improvement on the Restraint Scale was enhanced at six months and maintained at one-year follow-up.

With regard to the secondary outcomes of interest, no changes were demonstrated in depression, social adjustment, or blood pressure. Too few subjects complied with the request for repeated venipuncture, prohibiting useful analysis of the effects of education on blood values. There were significant reductions in scores on the bulimia and drive for thinness scales (as measured by the EDI). Bulimia scores continued to improve at six months and again at one year, while drive for thinness scores began to regress slightly at six months with slightly continued deterioration at one year. Weight and percent average weight did not change over the intervention period, had a slight increase at six months, and had returned to baseline at one-year follow-up.

Effect of Experiential Intervention

The Experiential group had a significantly greater impact on participants than the Education group. Both measures of self-esteem, and both scales of restrained eating pattern were significantly improved and the effect was maintained at six-month and one-year follow-up. Body dissatisfaction scores improved at the end of treatment but were not maintained at follow-up.

For the secondary outcome variables, levels of depression and social adjustment were significantly improved at posttest time but were not maintained at the follow-up. As in the Education group, both bulimia and drive for thinness scores were improved and maintained at six months, with regression in only the drive for thinness scores at one year. Weight, percent average weight, blood pressure and serum measures of fasting glucose, cholesterol, and lipids were unchanged by the intervention and at six-month posttest.

5

The Beyond Dieting Program: Discussion and Implications

This section discusses characteristics of the sample, the overall effects of the intervention (particularly in relation to self-esteem and body dissatisfaction), some hypotheses regarding the high levels of social maladjustment and reporting of symptoms of depression, and some implications of the findings.

EFFECTS OF THE INTERVENTION

The regression analysis indicated that group assignment was of greatest predictive power in explaining the results of this study. This was as expected for an intervention trial. Beyond the group effect, better results (that is, greater change in scores) were achieved by participants who entered with lower self-esteem according to the Janis and Field Feelings of Inadequacy scale, and higher restraint using Herman and Polivy's scale. These findings may indicate a regression to the mean, such that most participants simply reached a more normal level. Those women who were furthest from the norm at pretest had the greatest changes.

The Experiential group had a greater impact than the Education group. It is important to note, however, that education alone, had an effect. The exploration of cultural issues and information about normal eating and about set-point seemed to have a significant impact on the participants in both treatment groups. The added

115

benefit in the more intense group was attributed to more indivi-
dualized attention given to the participants about their eating patterns,
and to the cognitive and assertiveness exercises.

The Sample

In many ways, the women who responded to the general media
coverage, and subsequently agreed to participate were comparable
to clinically ill samples. Scores on both self-esteem scales and the
Restraint Scale matched those reported for patients with eating
disorders. Similarly, scores on the Weissman Social Adjustment Scale
were comparable to psychiatric outpatient samples of alcoholics and
schizophrenics (Weissman et al., 1978). Scores on the Depression
Scale were above the levels suggested to be a cutoff for mild
depression. In addition, scores on the three EDI subscales of body
dissatisfaction, bulimia, and drive for thinness matched the obese
sample (who were in a dieting group), surpassed the female controls,
but did not approach the eating disorder patients in the initial
validation of that instrument (Garner, Olmsted & Polivy, 1983).

This does not imply that all obese women are comparable to
these clinically ill groups. The literature review demonstrated that
obesity is not usually associated with the development of major
psychological disturbance. Participants in this study represent a subset
of the obese, who feel the need to enter into a program in order
to normalize eating patterns, as well as to improve self-esteem and
body dissatisfaction. Thus, obese women who judged themselves as
acceptable and who did not experience eating as a problem would
not display interest in this program.

Self-Esteem, Body Dissatisfaction and Restraint

As is evident from the literature review, the social pressure placed
on women to be thin, and the resulting bias and discrimination
experienced due to the deviant status of obesity in our culture,
undoubtedly results in low self-esteem, body dissatisfaction, and

restrained eating for some obese women. This was true for the current study sample. Van Strien and Bergers (1988) have hypothesized that low self-esteem and other personality disturbances may precede overeating and weight gain, but it is even more likely that there is a continuous interaction between overeating and psychological and social functioning.

The more intense intervention improved self-esteem and body dissatisfaction scores for the participants, but the latter were not maintained at follow-up. There were small, but significant correlations between the two self-esteem measures and body dissatisfaction at pretest. These disappeared at posttest, lending moderate support to the assumption that the intervention reduced the importance of body satisfaction in determining overall self-esteem. At the six-month follow-up, there was again a significant negative correlation between body dissatisfaction and self-esteem on the Rosenberg Scale, not with the Janis and Field Scale scores. This supports the notion that body dissatisfaction may have been decoupled from self-esteem, with some return to the baseline at follow-up.

In retrospect, it would have been useful to further test the concept of centrality, not just by correlations of body dissatisfaction with self-esteem, but with ratings of subjective importance of appearance as has been reported in some literature (Boldrick, 1983; Lerner, Karabenick & Stuart, 1973; Pliner, Chaiken & Flett, 1987). One woman who experienced an improvement from low self-esteem scores to the normal range as demonstrated (at follow-up) by her own statement that she was now able to separate dislike of her body from her overall self-esteem: "I feel that I am a capable individual, if not more capable than most. I am horribly overweight so it is this aspect of my life that I hate. I have most other things just right, except for this."

Heatherton, Polivy and Herman (Heatherton, 1986; Polivy, Heatherton & Herman, 1988) have studied the relationship among self-esteem and restraint and eating behavior in college women of normal weight. They found that self-esteem was not related to eating behavior in unrestrained women. However, in the restrained group, those with low self-esteem were more prone to disinhibition of their eating than those with high self-esteem. It is interesting to note that it was difficult to find restrained women with high self-esteem. These studies relate to the present study in that the obese women had high restraint scores and low self-esteem. If the findings can be generalized to obese women, one would expect the current study sample to also be easily disinhibited. That is, they may readily overeat after alcohol, stress, or when they have "blown their diets."

This hypothesis is supported by the scores on the bulimia scale of the Eating Disorder Inventory which are higher than those of female controls, and by the work by Telch and collegues (1988) who found that binge eating was significantly more prevalent as degree of obesity increased. Unfortunately, these data do not answer Heatherton's question of whether it is low self-esteem that causes restrained eaters to binge, whether binge eating results in low self-esteem, or whether it is a vicious cycle of both (Heatherton, 1986). However, as demonstrated in this study, both are amenable to change. Self-esteem and level of restraint were significantly improved and maintained in this study by the more intense intervention.

Social Maladjustment:

The majority of the women in this study had been obese as children or adolescents, and had mean scores on the Weissmann Scale that indicated poor social adjustment. Stunkard and Mendelson (1967) have described disturbances in body image in the obese to be associated with self-consciousness and with impaired social functioning. They have found that body image disturbance arose among emotionally disturbed persons whose obesity began prior to adult life and whose families did not value their obesity. This disturbance was not affected by weight reduction but was favorably altered by long-term psychotherapy. They did not report if social functioning was improved along with body image disturbance.

The results of this study show the Experiential group experienced only a transient improvement in social adjustment scores. One would expect that if self-esteem scores were maintained, social adjustment would show a concomitant maintenance. This did not occur in the present study. To a large extent, the Weissman Scale is based on social interaction. It is probable that even though self-esteem improved, subjects' families, coworkers, peers, and society generally still look negatively upon these women and their obesity. Since their interactions do not improve, social adjustment does not show a change.

Depression

There are several possible explanations for the unusually high levels of depressive symptoms reported by this obese sample. One possibility is that depression is related to bulimic symptoms that were undiagnosed in these subjects. Prather and Williamson (1988), compared 16 obese patients who presented themselves at an eating disorder clinic with 16 non-dieting obese women. The clinic population had significantly higher depression scores as rated by the Beck Depression Inventory. These authors concluded that it may be that depression is one of the most important problems for the obese person seeking treatment (p. 182), and should be a screening and referral component of any weight loss program. Furthermore, they postulated that, since depression is the most prevalent associated feature of bulimia, depression in the obese may be a symptom of bulimia.

Support for the relationship between binge eating and obesity has been reported by Keefe et al. (1984). They found that 23% of 44 women enrolled in a behavioral treatment program for obesity met DSM-III criteria for current bulimia. Further, Hudson and colleagues (1988) reported that 17% of their obese community sample met the same criteria. In contrast to the normal weight bulimic samples, the obese infrequently used self-induced vomiting to purge; thus they were less effective in controlling weight gain following a binge episode. It is a weakness of the present study that no clinical evaluation was done to screen the participants for eating disorders beyond self and family physician report.

Depressive symptoms may also be experienced by this obese group as a result of feeling that one does not fit society's expectation of thinness in women. Rosen, Gross and Vara (1987) studied the relationship between depression scores on the Beck Depression Inventory and adolescents' attempts to lose or gain weight. Females had lower depression scores if they were actually underweight than if at normal weight or overweight, whereas males had lower scores if they were overweight. This lends further support to the notion that obese females bear the burden of social consequences of deviance from the cultural norm and may explain why the depression scores in the present study were in the mildly depressed range.

Noles and colleagues (1985) found support for the relationship between self-rated attractiveness and depression. Over two hundred college students completed the CES-D Scale, were videotaped, rated themselves on a scale of physical attractiveness, and then were rated by reliable viewers on the same dimension. Depressed subjects were less satisfied with their bodies and saw themselves as less physically attractive than nondepressed subjects. These groups did not differ on observer-rated attractiveness. Interestingly, there was a substantial positive distortion among nondepressed subjects, who rated themselves as more attractive than did the observer-ratings. This study does not answer the question of causation: Does depression cause negative self-rating of attractiveness or vice versa?

During the intervention, it was clear from anecdotal information that participants saw themselves as unattractive. As in the college students from the study by Noles, Cash and Winstead (1985), the self-rating of unattractiveness may help account for these "mild depression" scores.

The Experiential intervention had a short-term impact on improving depression scores. Both interventions reduced scores to levels at, or below, the cutoff for "mild depression," which may be a clinically significant change regardless of its statistical meaning.

Physiological Variables

Weight, blood pressure and available serum results indicated that physiological measures did not deteriorate as subjects normalized scores on self-esteem, body dissatisfaction, restraint, symptoms of depression, social adjustment, bulimia, and drive for thinness. This is an important finding for clinicians treating obese patients who are diagnosed with hypertension and diabetes mellitus. Perhaps patients should not be admonished to reduce weight for management of these conditions; rather, they should be encouraged to eat normally and exercise in moderation. The stability of the physiological measures in the face of improving psychosocial measures is important. Unlike dieting, which is associated with deteriorating scores on depression, restraint, self-esteem, bulimia, and drive for thinness, the non-dieting intervention was associated with improvement on the same measures.

LIMITATIONS OF THE STUDY

It is important to keep in mind the weaknesses of this study when discussing and interpreting results. They include:

1. High drop-out rates at the time of the six-month follow-up. This may contribute to the finding of a lack of maintenance of effect at follow-up as the sample size may have become too small to have the power to show a significant difference. There was an even greater drop-out at one-year follow-up.
2. The lack of a control group at six months and one-year follow-up. This limits the relevant analysis for the follow-up period.
3. The lack of clinical evaluation screening for eating disorders. It is impossible to estimate the proportion of the sample with eating disorders, but the literature review gives evidence for increased binge eating in the obese. Overall bulimia scores for both intervention groups improved. However, a clinical

evaluation might have permitted sub-analysis of a clinical and nonclinical population.

4. Experimenter bias. The same person solicited participation, administered tests, and delivered the intervention. Close relationships developed with participants over the 12-week program and this may have led them to score in a particular fashion in order to please the experimenter. Simply knowing that they were participating in a study could influence participants' responses, so that the two intervention groups, but not the control group, may show changes in scores.

5. For the most part, the "correct response" is evident in the questionnaires, allowing participants to choose the socially desirable response, which could lead to inflation of scores. A social desirability scale could have been included. However, if this bias was operant, it had an inconsistent effect, since scores improved on the restraint scales (where the socially desirable response is less evident) and self-esteem, but did not significantly improve in social adjustment or depression. Therefore, it is less obvious that social desirability was producing the improvement in scores.

6. Both interventions were conducted by the author. This could have affected results because the therapists' preference for an intervention may have been communicated in subtle ways.

7. No attempt was made to match the client with the intervention. This was a controlled trial to compare results of the two interventions, not for specificity of treatments.

8. The women who agreed to participate probably were not a representative sample of the population of all obese women. A bias was introduced in terms of appeal to respondents—the responders were those who identified that they needed to do something (other than entering another weight loss program) about their unhappiness with their bodies. Thus, women who were reasonably satisfied with themselves or who had a strong belief that they could/would lose weight did not enter the program.

9. Test scores were not available on drop-outs from this study. If they could have been obtained, overall results may have been less positive, as it is likely that they stopped coming because the program was not meeting their needs.

10. The follow-up period was short. It is extremely important to follow this group to one-year posttreatment and beyond to ensure that any changes maintained at six months have not been diminished.

SUGGESTIONS FOR IMPROVING THE INTERVENTIONS

Overall, the more intense Experiential intervention was more effective in producing positive change in obese subjects. For this reason, it is recommended that it is the Experiential intervention that should be administered in the future.

Education alone resulted in significant change in the area of restraint and was approaching significance in improving self-esteem. There are methods that may enhance the effect of an education program. For example, the provision of a participant's manual, with readings and exercises to do at home, should be tested to determine whether it would enhance the effect of the education component. An alternative would be to evaluate a stepped program of intervention, starting first with education, followed by the more intensive intervention (for those who needed it as determined by lesser change in target outcomes), followed by individual psychotherapy as indicated.

With regard to changes in the Experiential intervention, it is recommended that the same intervention be evaluated with an obese person as group leader. The presence of a positive role model may possibly potentiate the effectiveness of the intervention. The current study was done by a normal-weight group leader who had never herself experienced the process of change from the diet mentality to the non-diet approach.

It is also recommended that participants attend "booster" sessions on a monthly basis and that this be evaluated to determine if it improves maintenance of change in scores on social adjustment, body dissatisfaction and depression. Of particular importance is the focus on dealing with the grieving process associated with the loss of the dream to be thin, which was observed in the participants toward the end of the 12 weeks. In addition, it is recommended that information sessions for "supportive others" be included, similar to Brownell and Wadden's (1986) suggestion for obesity treatment, and evaluated for impact on social adjustment. Of potentially greater impact would be to have spouses or friends attend the entire intervention, perhaps with exercises developed specifically for them.

Many people who phoned NEDIC and attended the information sessions were below the weight criteria. The intervention could be modified and tested with normal weight women who are concerned about body weight and shape, and who wish to change their eating patterns. Over the two-year period, about 20 phone calls came from men who wished to participate in the program. The effectiveness of male or coeducational groups could also be tested.

IMPLICATIONS FOR OTHER RESEARCH

This study constituted an efficacy trial of interventions that could be an alternative to dieting in obese women. Now that efficacy has been established for the Experiential intervention, it would be useful to compare a diet versus non-diet approach, where participants who were willing to do "something" about their weight would be randomized to groups and compared on the same outcomes of self-esteem, restraint, body dissatisfaction, depression, social adjustment, weight and, particularly, the physiological variables. As noted in the literature review, there is considerable controversy over whether or not dieting improves or produces low self-esteem, depression, weight gain, high blood pressure, and abnormal serum levels of glucose, cholesterol, and lipids. The randomized trial just described would answer some of those questions and follow logically from the current study.

CONCLUSIONS

Chapter 2 described a sample of obese women who, at pretest time, had scores on self-esteem, restraint, depression, and social adjustment that were abnormal when compared with the norms reported in the literature. This study established that the 12-week group intervention described in Chapter 3 can be effective in improving self-esteem, encouraging a restrained pattern of eating and, in the short term, improving body dissatisfaction, depression, and social adjustment without change in weight or blood pressure. Further testing is required to establish generalizability to women of other weight ranges, younger females, and men. The intervention might be further strengthened by inclusion of a participants' manual of readings and exercises to support group activity, by attendance at booster sessions, or by involvement of supportive others.

Further work is needed in order to determine how best to counsel patient and nonpatient populations about dieting versus non-dieting. Given the dismal results of weight-reduction attempts reported in this literature review, it seems unwise to promote dieting in the obese who are currently free from hypertension, hypercholesterolemia, or hyperglycemia. If those risk factors exist, a suggested intervention is to take a careful diet history to determine what kind/how many diets the person has already tried. A weight reduction diet is unlikely to be effective if several previous attempts have been unsuccessful. In every case, exercise may be more beneficial than weight reduction through caloric restriction.

The intervention described had some positive effects, but it is anticipated that cultural change, perhaps through widespread community education, is necessary to reduce the emotional burden of body disparagement, poor self-esteem, and social discrimination experienced by some obese and normal-weight women who perceive their deviance from the stringent standards for thinness in women.

This program presents a viable alternative to ongoing diet attempts for obese women. It resulted in better emotional health for the women who were part of the evaluation. It is hoped that health professionals will take the outline presented in Chapter 3 and adapt it to their style and the needs of the particular group involved. In this way, we will promote the individual and societal change necessary to reach the future goal of acceptance of the whole range of body shapes and sizes, and of valuing individuals for their abilities and personalities rather than for body shape.

Appendix A

Information Sheet

There is growing evidence that one's body weight is determined by biology and is highly resistant to reduction or maintenance of a reduced weight. It is now less clear that being overweight increases your risk of becoming ill. Yet the media and culture in general place a high premium on being thin. Consequently, many women spend countless dollars, hours, and energy striving for that unrealistic ideal.

Dieting, while showing immediate, short-term results, is difficult to maintain, and eventually the body responds by mechanisms that maintain higher weight than would be expected from the low intake. In addition, dieting has been associated in some people with many unpleasant and unhealthy side effects such as fatigue, irritability, depression, and eating disorders (e.g., bulimia). The usual result is that the dieter becomes discouraged and gives up the food restriction for a period of time. Any weight loss is quickly restored and the woman feels a level of failure and reduced self-esteem. This cycle is repeated many times in the lives of overweight women. This "yo-yo" effect may be more hazardous to health than maintaining a higher but constant weight.

This study is designed to evaluate the effects of a program for overweight women which is aimed at establishing normal eating patterns and improving their self-esteem. It will also evaluate the effects of the program on blood pressure and the amounts of fats and sugar in the blood. You should not participate in this study if you are pregnant, or if you have a diagnosed

127

medical or psychiatric problem. The expected benefit (if any) is that you will gain useful information. There are no anticipated risks.

This study has three phases. You are invited to participate in all phases, but you are also welcome to complete some of the phases and not others. You are free to withdraw from the study at any time.

Phase 1.

Your participation would consist of completing a packet of questionnaires about yourself and your style of eating. Your blood pressure, height, and weight will be taken. You will also be requested to take the information letter and consent form to your physician to sign. He or she will be asked to take a blood sample from you as well. We want to ensure that there are no medical reasons why you should not participate in this program.

Phase 2.

Your participation would consist of attending a 1- to 2-hour session, once per week for 12 weeks. The sessions will cover the information presented in the introduction above—the biology of weight regulation, the effects of dieting, the cultural pressure on women to be thin. The small group format will be used to allow you to ask questions. These sessions will be held at the Health League of Canada offices, Toronto. At the completion of the 12 sessions, you will again be asked to complete the questionnaires, and have your blood sample, weight, and pressure assessed.

Phase 3.

Your participation would consist of completing a packet of questionnaires, having your blood sample, weight and blood pressure assessed six and 12 months after completion of the sessions.

In order to carefully evaluate the effects of this program, some participants will be asked to wait until the program is offered the second time. At this time, they will again complete the questionnaires and begin the 12-week series of sessions.

Any information you provide in any phase of the study will be kept completely confidential. You will be asked to put your name on a cover sheet only and not on the questionnaires themselves. When you return a questionnaire, the cover sheet will be immediately removed and a code number will be placed on the questionnaire. The list matching names with the code numbers will be kept only by the principal investigator, to be destroyed by her when the study is finished. The results of the study will be reported in such a way that individuals cannot be identified.

Your cooperation in any phase does not in any way commit you to participation in any of the other phases.

Thank you for your cooperation.

Consent Form

The study of Dr. David Garner and Donna Ciliska concerning self-esteem in overweight women has been explained to me. Any questions I have asked have been answered to my satisfaction. I have been informed that study participation is voluntary. I understand the benefits, risks and discomforts (if any) of joining the above study. I am aware that I can withdraw from the study at any time. I know that I may ask now, or in the future any questions that I have about the study. Any information that I provide will be kept strictly confidential. Questionnaires will be coded by number. The list matching codes with names will be accessible only to the principal investigator and will be destroyed when the study is finished. No information will be released that would disclose personal identity.

1. I agree to complete the initial package of questionnaires, and have weight, height, blood pressure taken, and to have my physician take a blood sample for glucose and lipids and report it to the investigator.

Yes ____   No ____

2. I agree to attend a series of weekly sessions for 12 weeks about the effects of dieting, biology of weight regulation, and factors related to self-esteem, and would be willing to complete the same questionnaires and physical assessment measures for the purpose of evaluating the sessions. I understand that commencement of this series may be delayed by 12 weeks to allow for thorough evaluation of this program.

Yes ____   No ____

3. I agree to be contacted six and twelve months after completion of the program to complete the same questionnaires and physical assessment measures.

Yes ____   No ____

Name _____ Signature _____
            Please Print

Thank you very much for your cooperation.

Physician's Consent Request

Dear Dr. ————————————————

We are requesting your consent for your patient ————————————— to participate in a new program and its evaluation. This program of Dr. David Garner and Donna Ciliska is a 12-week (one to two hours/week) group intervention for obese women aimed at improving self-esteem and establishing normal eating habits.

There is a growing evidence that one's body weight is determined by biology and is highly resistant to reduction or maintenance of a reduced weight. It is now less clear that being overweight alone increases health risks. Overweight women go through cycles of attempted weight loss by food restriction, followed by small weight loss, frustration with plateaus from depressed metabolic rate and quick regain. The result is a sense of failure and reduced self-esteem.

This program will be primarily educational concerning nutrition, eating management, the biology of weight control, and the effects of dieting on nutrition and emotions. It will sensitize women to the arbitrariness of the cultural emphasis on body shape.

A package of questionnaires related to diet history, self-esteem and self concept will be given to the participants as a pretest, posttest and 6 and 12-month posttest. There will be a wait-list control group for purposes of careful evaluation. Therefore, the start of the program will be delayed by 12 weeks for some women. All measures will be coded and will remain strictly confidential. The participants are free to withdraw at any time.

We wish to exclude from this program any patients who are pregnant or have a diagnosed medical or psychiatric problem. The expected benefit (if any) is that useful information will be gained by the participants. There are no anticipated risks.

If your patient is not excluded on the above grounds, please sign the attached consent and arrange for her to have blood samples taken for fasting blood glucose and lipids. We wish to see if these measures are affected by normalizing eating patterns. Please report these on the enclosed card and return in the stamped, addressed envelope.

Physician's Consent Form

I consent to have my patient _____
(patient's name) take part in a study by Dr. David Garner and Donna
Ciliska, of the effects of a group intervention program on the self-esteem
of obese women, as described on the attached form.

This patient is not pregnant and does not have a major medical or
psychiatric problem diagnosed.

I understand that written consent has been obtained from the patient.
Participation in the study is voluntary and the participant can withdraw
at any time. For some women, commencement of the program may be
delayed by 12 weeks if they have been randomized to the control group.

Any information obtained will be coded, and kept strictly confidential.
No information will be released or printed that would disclose personal
identity.

_____

Signature of Physician

_____

Date

Appendix B

ANALYSIS OF VARIANCE
(ANOVA) TABLES

TABLE B.1
Three-Factor Eating Questionnaire—Overall Scores

	Assessment Time									Pre- Posttest Comparison		Post- 6 Months		Pre- 6 Months	
	Pretest			Posttest			6 Months								
Group	N	M	SD	N	M	SD	N	M	SD	F	P	F	P	F	P
Education	42	29.54	6.48	33	26.0	7.46	24	23.21	7.20	4.82	0.0313	1.9985	0.1631	6.6	0.0021
Experiential	49	32.09	5.96	39	25.01	7.59	28	23.22	8.66	24.0052	0.0000	0.8007	.3742	17.02	0.0000
Control	45	31.54	5.75	27	29.51	6.8	—	—	—	1.8512	.178	—	—	—	—
Intergroup Comparison															
F	2.1676														
P	0.1184														

TABLE B.2
Three-Factor Eating Questionnaire—Cognitive Control

	Assessment Time									Pre- Posttest Comparison		Post- 6 Months		Pre- 6 Months	
	Pretest			Posttest			6 Months								
Group	N	M	SD	N	M	SD	N	M	SD	F	P	F	P	F	P
Education	42	8.60	4.40	33	7.74	3.77	24	7.82	3.49	0.7891	0.3773	0.0071	0.9329	0.5131	0.6003
Experiential	49	9.61	3.89	39	7.39	3.74	28	6.98	3.68	7.3264	0.0082	0.1955	0.6598	5.729	0.0043
Control	45	9.38	3.99	27	8.58	3.54	—	—	—	0.7522	0.3888	—	—	—	—
Intergroup Comparison															
F	0.7499														
P	0.4744														

135

TABLE B.3
Three-Factor Eating Questionnaire—Susceptibility to Hunger

Group	Assessment Time									Pre- Posttest Comparison		Post- 6 Months		Pre- 6 Months	
	Pretest			Posttest			6 Months								
	N	M	SD	N	M	SD	N	M	SD	F	P	F	P	F	P
Education	43	8.57	3.57	33	7.44	3.36	24	6.05	3.91	1.9817	0.1634	2.0795	0.1550	3.8662	0.0242
Experiential	49	9.22	3.06	39	7.50	3.32	28	7.11	6.62	6.4008	0.0132	1.849	0.6686	4.45	0.0138
Control	45	8.98	3.28	27	8.52	3.45	—	—	—	—	—	—	—	—	—
Intergroup Comparison															
F	0.4478														
P	0.6400														

TABLE B.4
Three-Factor Eating Questionnaire—Disinhibition of Control

Group	Assessment Time									Pre- Posttest Comparison		Post- 6 Months		Pre- 6 Months	
	Pretest			Posttest			6 Months								
	N	M	SD	N	M	SD	N	M	SD	F	P	F	P	F	P
Education	43	12.39	2.58	33	10.82	3.25	24	9.34	3.90	5.54	0.0213	2.4778	0.1249	7.446	0.0010
Experiential	49	13.25	2.28	39	10.13	3.27	28	9.14	4.07	27.8896	0.0000	1.2183	0.2738	19.01	0.0000
Control	45	13.18	2.04	27	12.41	2.93	—	—	—	1.7305	0.1926	—	—	—	—
Intergroup Comparison															
F	1.9143														
P	0.1515														

TABLE B.5
Glucose

Group	Pretest			Posttest			6 Months			Pre-Posttest Comparison		Post-6 Months		Pre-6 Months	
	N	M	SD	N	M	SD	N	M	SD	F	P	F	P	F	P
				Assessment Time											
Education	26	5.35	0.67	10	5.44	0.55	4	5.25	0.1430	0.7077	—	—	—	—	—
Experiential	32	5.29	0.84	16	4.9	1.43	12	5.34	0.43	1.55006	0.2194	1.1911	0.2851	1.0932	0.3241
Control	10	6.05	0.92	—			—			—		—		—	

Intergroup Comparison
F 1.4544
P 0.2410

TABLE B.6
Cholesterol

Group	Pretest			Posttest			6 Months			Pre-Posttest Comparison		Post-6 Months		Pre-6 Months	
	N	M	SD	N	M	SD	N	M	SD	F	P	F	P	F	P
				Assessment Time											
Education	26	5.36	0.92	11	5.82	1.09	4	5.47	0.92	1.0659	0.3075	—	—	—	—
Experiential	29	5.60	0.99	17	5.73	0.89	12	5.73	0.88	2.0743	0.1837	0.3808	0.5424	0.7189	0.4918
Control	10	4.73	0.71	—			—			—		—		—	

Intergroup Comparison
F 3.2348
P 0.0461

TABLE B.7
High-Density Lipoproteins (HDL) Cholesterol

| | Assessment Time | | | | | | | | | Pre- Posttest Comparison | | Post- 6 Months | | Pre- 6 Months | |
| | Pretest | | | Posttest | | | 6 Months | | | | | | | | |
Group	N	M	SD	N	M	SD	N	M	SD	F	P	F	P	F	P
Education	21	1.31	0.48	9	1.64	0.32	4	5.25	0.78	1.0313	0.3186	—	—	—	—
Experiential	20	1.30	0.26	14	1.24	0.22	12	5.34	0.43	0.5517	0.463	1.2125	0.2839	1.404	0.2578
Control	6	1.24	0.28	—	—	—	—	—	—	—	—	—	—	—	—

Intergroup Comparison
F   0.092
P   0.939

TABLE B.8
Triglycerides

| | Assessment Time | | | | | | | | | Pre- Posttest Comparison | | Post- 6 Months | | Pre- 6 Months | |
| | Pretest | | | Posttest | | | 6 Months | | | | | | | | |
Group	N	M	SD	N	M	SD	N	M	SD	F	P	F	P	F	P
Education	27	2.05	1.9	11	1.81	0.73	4	2.23	1.48	0.1653	0.6862	—	—	—	—
Experiential	31	1.64	1.5	17	1.80	0.82	12	2.34	1.59	2.525	0.1189	0.0549	0.8165	1.2719	0.2881
Control	10	2.94	0.9	—	—	—	—	—	—	—	—	—	—	—	—

Intergroup Comparison
F   1.9924
P   0.1447

TABLE B.9
Weissman Social Adjustment Scale

Group	Pretest			Posttest			6 Months			Pre- Posttest Comparison		Post- 6 Months		Pre- 6 Months	
	N	M	SD	N	M	SD	N	M	SD	F	P	F	P	F	P
Education	45	2.04	0.36	38	1.94	0.33	24	1.84	0.33	1.7553	0.1889	1.3072	0.2574	2.7415	0.0691
Experiential	47	2.0	0.38	42	1.82	0.37	28	1.85	0.36	4.6078	0.0346	0.1140	0.7367	2.6190	0.0773
Control	45	2.27	0.54	27	2.1	0.49	—	—	—	1.8037	0.1836	—		—	

Intergroup Comparison
F 5.1735
P 0.0069

Control significantly different from intervention groups

TABLE B.10
Center for Epidemiologic Studies—Depression Scale

Group	Pretest			Posttest			6 Months			Pre- Posttest Comparison		Post- 6 Months		Pre- 6 Months	
	N	M	SD	N	M	SD	N	M	SD	F	P	F	P	F	P
Education	44	17.70	10.32	35	16.54	8.38	23	15.96	11.40	0.2907	0.5913	0.0509	0.8223	0.2690	0.7647
Experiential	49	17.70	10.27	41	12.20	11.01	26	14.08	9.923	4.5770	0.0352	0.5008	0.4817	2.4035	0.0950
Control	46	21.93	13.14	26	19.23	9.88	—			0.8239	0.3646	—		—	

Intergroup Comparison
F 2.591
P 0.08

TABLE B.11
Eating Disorder Inventory—Bulimia Scale

| | Assessment Time | | | | | | | | | | | | Pre- Posttest Comparison | | Post- 6 Months | |
| | Pretest | | | Posttest | | | 6 Months | | | 1 Year | | | | | | |
Measure/Group	N	M	SD	N	M	SD	N	M	SD	N	M	SD	F	P	F	P
Education	45	4.24	3.55	35	2.11	3.50	24	2.07	3.06	19	1.32	1.86	7.17	0.009	0.0026	0.957
Experiential	49	6.50	4.45	36	2.43	2.41	27	3.22	4.24	17	2.76	3.11	24.80	0.0001	0.8900	0.3492
Control	45	7.46	5.06	27	5.89	5.44	—	—	—	—	—	—	1.53	0.2206	—	—

TABLE B.12
Eating Disorder Inventory—Drive for Thinness Scale

| | Assessment Time | | | | | | | | | | | | Pre- Posttest Comparison | | Post- 6 Months | |
| | Pretest | | | Posttest | | | 6 Months | | | 1 Year | | | | | | |
Measure/Group	N	M	SD	N	M	SD	N	M	SD	N	M	SD	F	P	F	P
Education	44	7.86	5.43	35	4.40	4.49	24	5.83	5.48	19	6.0	5.58	9.24	0.0032	1.2152	0.2749
Experiential	49	10.41	5.81	36	4.83	4.68	27	4.50	5.31	17	6.0	6.46	22.43	0.0001	0.0698	0.7925
Control	45	11.96	5.94	27	11.26	5.56	—	—	—	—	—	—	0.2623	0.6101	—	—

Appendix C

CORRELATIONS OF SELF-ESTEEM WITH
BODY DISSATISFACTION BY GROUP

TABLE C.1

Correlations of Self-Esteem and Body Dissatisfaction by Group

	Janis & Field	Rosenberg	Body Dissatisfaction
Pretest			
Education Group (*n*=41):			
Janis & Field	1.000	−0.7716**	0.2370
Rosenberg	−0.7716**	1.000	−0.2906
Body Dissatisfaction	0.2370	−0.2906	1.000
Experiential Group (*n*=47):			
Janis & Field	1.000	−0.8422**	0.3884*
Rosenberg	−0.8422**	1.000	−0.2814
Body Dissatisfaction	0.3884*	−0.2814	1.000
Control Group (*n*=42):			
Janis & Field	1.000	−0.8282**	0.3442
Rosenberg	−0.8282**	1.000	−0.1954
Body Dissatisfaction	0.3442	−0.1954	1.000
Posttest			
Education Group (*n*=33):			
Janis & Field	1.000	−0.7578**	0.0932
Rosenberg	−0.7578**	1.000	−0.1820
Body Dissatisfaction	0.0932	−0.1820	1.000
Experiential Group (*n*=35):			
Janis & Field	1.000	−0.5755**	0.1387
Rosenberg	−0.5755**	1.000	−0.2410
Body Dissatisfaction	0.1387	−0.2410	1.000
Six-Month follow-up			
Education Group (*n*=23):			
Janis & Field	1.000	−0.8316**	0.2213
Rosenberg	−0.8316**	1.000	−0.4158
Body Dissatisfaction	0.2213	−0.4158	1.000
Experiential Group (*n*=25):			
Janis & Field	1.000	−0.7901**	0.3318
Rosenberg	−0.7901**	1.000	−0.2041
Body Dissatisfaction	0.3318	−0.2041	1.000

*Indicates significance at $p < 0.01$
**Indicates significance at $p < 0.001$

Appendix D

BEYOND DIETING—PROCESS EVALUATION

This form has been devised for you to anonymously give feedback to the program developers. Please keep in mind that others will be participating in the program after you. We would like to make it as beneficial as possible. Therefore, we look forward to your honest comments.

Circle the number for each aspect of the course content that *best* describes how you felt about the session.

	Cannot remember, or absent	Uninteresting/ useless	Interesting/ useful somewhat	very
Cultural pressures to be thin	0	1	2	3
Prejudice against obesity	0	1	2	3
Effects of dieting on mood	0	1	2	3
Effects of dieting on eating behavior	0	1	2	3
Makeup session	0	1	2	3
Colors/styles session	0	1	2	3
Explanation of set point	0	1	2	3
Reasons for normal eating	0	1	2	3
Myths regarding health risks	0	1	2	3
Recommendations regarding exercise	0	1	2	3
Discussion of causes of obesity	0	1	2	3
Discussion of myth of personality disturbance in obese	0	1	2	3
Rating of overall program	0	1	2	3

How would you rate the group spirit?

	Committed/supportive	Neutral	Cool/uninvolved
Size of group:	too big	O.K.	too small
Amount of time for discussion/ questions?	too much	O.K.	too little
Length of the program (in weeks)?	too long	O.K.	too short

Please rate that group leader on the following qualities:

Understanding of issues regarding obesity	good	O.K.	needs improvement
Enthusiasm	good	O.K.	needs improvement
Ability to hold your interest	good	O.K.	needs improvement

Do you have any suggestions or comments for this person?

What aspect of the program had the greatest effect on your attitudes or behavior?

On which topics or aspects of the program would you like to see more time spent?

Do you have any other suggestions for how the program could be improved? (for example, group size, setting, time)

Any other comments would be appreciated.

Appendix E

ANNOTATED BIBLIOGRAPHY

Overweight as a Health Risk Factor

Andres, R. (1980). Effect of obesity on total mortality. *International Journal of Obesity, 4,* 381–386. Review of several studies showing that obesity is not a risk for overall mortality.

Brunzell, J.D. (1984). Are all obese patients at risk for cardiovascular disease? *International Journal of Obesity, 8,* 571–578. Supports hypothesis: a significant proportion of risk of obesity for coronary artery disease is mediated through specific familial disorders which are associated with both obesity and premature coronary artery disease.

Fitzgerald, F.T. (1981). The problem of obesity. *Annual Review of Medicine, 33,* 221–231.

Hibscher, J.A. & Herman, C.P. (1977). Obesity, dieting, and the expression of "obese" characteristics. *Journal of Comparative and Physiological Psychology, 91,* 374–380. Free fatty acids were a function of dieting, not obesity, in college females (obese, normal, and underweight).

Simopoulos, A.P. (1985). The health implication of overweight and obesity. *Nutrition Review, 43,* 33–40. Review of Framingham and several other studies. Careful look at the evidence presented in the paper contradicts conclusions of this review that overweight people die earlier and that obesity is a single independent risk factor for cardiovascular disease.

Simopoulos, A.P. & Van Itallie, T.B. (1984). Body weight, health, and longevity. *Annals of Internal Medicine, 100,* 285–295. Same paper as above with a better review than Simopoulos (1985).

Sorlie, P., Gordon, T. & Kannel, W.B. (1980). Body build and mortality—The Framingham Study. *Journal of the American Medical Association, 243,* 1828–1831. Women who are 5'3" to 5'6", 115–195 pounds, have no differences in mortality risk as weight increases.

Wooley, S.C. & Wooley, O.W. (1984). Should obesity be treated at all? In A.J. Stunkard & E. Stellar (Eds.), *Eating and Its Disorders*. New York: Raven Press. Presents evidence that there is biological control over weight, weight loss programs are ineffective, lack of clear evidence that obesity alone is a health risk.

For a more readable review see:
Polivy, J. & Herman, C.P. (1983). *Breaking the Diet Habit*. New York: Basic Books, 54–74.

References

Adler, A. (1929). *The Practice and Theory of Individual Psychology*. London: Routledge & Kegan Paul.

Albanes, D., Jones, D. Y., Micozzi, M. S. & Mattson, M. E. (1987). Associations between smoking and body weight in the US population: Analysis of NHANES II. *American Journal of Public Health, 77,* 439–444.

Allbeck, P., Hallberg, D. & Espmark, S. (1976). Body-image—An apparatus for measuring disturbances in estimation of size and shape. *Journal of Psychosomatic Medicine, 20,* 583–589.

Allen, J. D. (1988). Knowing what to weigh: Women's self-care activities related to weight. *Advances in Nursing Science, 11,* 47–60.

Allon, N. (1975). The stigma of obesity in everyday life. In G. Bray (Ed.), *Obesity in Perspective*. Washington: Government Printing Office.

Andres, R. (1980). Effect of obesity on total mortality. *International Journal of Obesity, 4,* 381–386.

Askevold, F. (1975). Measuring body image. *Psychotherapy and Psychosomatics, 26,* 71–75.

Barocas, R. & Vance, F. L. (1974). Physical appearance and personal adjustment counseling. *Journal of Counseling Psychology, 21,* 96–100.

Bass, M., Buck, C. & Donner, A. (1985). Does obesity in men reduce the risks of hypertension? *Clinical and Investigative Medicine, 8,* A131.

Beck, A. T., Rush, A. J., Shaw, B. F. & Emery, G. (1979). *Cognitive Therapy of Depression*. New York: Guilford.

Beck, A. T., Ward, C. H., Mendelson, M., Mock, J. & Erbaugh, J. (1961). An inventory for measuring depression. *Archives of General Psychiatry, 4,* 561–571.

Bennett, W. & Gurin, J. (1982). *The Dieter's Dilemma*. New York: Basic Books.

Benson, H. (1975). *The Relaxation Response*. New York: William Morrow.

Ben-Tovim, D. I. (1988). DSM-III, draft DSM-III-R, and the diagnosis and prevalence of bulimia in Australia. *American Journal of Psychiatry, 145,* 1000–1002.

149

Berscheid, E., Walster, E. & Bohrnstedt, G. (1973). The happy American body: A survey report. *Psychology Today, 1,* (November), 119–131.

Bitsch, M. & Skrumsager, B. K. (1987). Femoxetene in the treatment of obese patients in general practice. A randomized group comparative study with placebo. *International Journal of Obesity, 11,* 183–190.

Bjorntorp, P. (1976). Exercise in the treatment of obesity. *Clinics in Endocrinology and Metabolism, 5,* 431–453.

Bjorntorp, P., Bergman, H. & Vanauskas, E. (1969). Plasma free fatty acid turnover in obesity. *Acta Medica Scandinavica, 185,* 351–356.

Boldrick, L. M. (1983). Psychological centrality of physical attributes: A reexamination of the relationship between subjective importance and self esteem. *Journal of Psychology, 115,* 97–102.

Booth, D. A. (1980). Acquired behavior controlling energy intake and output. In Stunkard, A. J. (Ed.), *Obesity.* Toronto: Saunders.

Borjeson, M. (1976). The aetiology of obesity in children. *Acta Pediatrica Scandinavia, 65,* 279–287.

Bouchard, C. (1986). Genetics of body fat, energy expenditure and adipose tissue metabolism. In E. M. Berry, S. H. Blondheim, H. E. Eliahou & E. Shafrir (Eds.), *Recent Advances in Obesity Research: V* (pp. 16–25). London: John Libbey.

Bray, G. A. (1969). Effect of caloric restriction on energy expenditure in obese patients. *Lancet, 2,* 397–398.

Bray, G. A. (1978). Definition, measurement and classification of the syndromes of obesity. *International Journal of Obesity, 2,* 99–112.

Bray, G. A. (1985). Obesity: Definition, diagnosis and disadvantages. *Medical Journal of Australia, 142,* S2–S8.

Brook, C. G. D., Huntley, R. M. C. & Slack, J. (1975). Influence of heredity and environment in determination of skinfold thickness in children. *British Medical Journal, 2,* 719–721.

Brownell, K. D. (1984). Behavioral, psychological, and environmental predictors of obesity and success at weight reduction. *International Journal of Obesity, 8,* 543–550.

Brownell, K. D., Greenwood, M. R. C., Stellar, E. & Shrager, E. E. (1986). The effects of repeated cycles of weight loss and regain in rats. *Physiology and Behavior, 38,* 459–464.

Brownell, K. D. & Stunkard, A. J. (1980). Physical activity in the development and control of obesity. In A. J. Stunkard (Ed.), *Obesity* (pp. 300–324). Philadelphia: Saunders.

Brownell, K. D. & Wadden, T. A. (1986). Behavior therapy for obesity: Modern approaches and better results. In K. D. Brownell, & J. P. Foreyt (Eds.),

Handbook of Eating Disorders: Physiology, Psychology, and Treatment of Obesity, Anorexia, and Bulimia (pp. 180–197). New York: Basic Books.

Bruch, H. (1973). *Eating Disorders: Obesity, Anorexia Nervosa, and the Person Within*. New York: Basic Books.

Bruch, H. (1978). *The Golden Cage*. Cambridge: Harvard University Press.

Brunzell, J. D. (1984). Are all obese patients at risk for cardiovascular disease? *International Journal of Obesity, 8,* 571–578.

Butters, J. W. & Cash, T. F. (1987). Cognitive-behavioral treatment of women's body-image dissatisfaction. *Journal of Consulting and Clinical Psychology, 55,* 889–897.

Canada Fitness Survey. (1981) Government of Canada, Fitness and Amateur Sport. Ottawa.

Canada Fitness Survey. (1985) Government of Canada, Fitness and Amateur Sport. Ottawa.

Canning, H. & Mayer, J. (1966). Obesity—its possible effects on college admissions. *New England Journal of Medicine, 275,* 1172–1174.

Cash, T. F. (1985). Physical appearance and mental health. In J. A. Graham & A. Kligman (Eds.), *The Psychology of Cosmetic Treatments* (pp. 196–216). New York: Praeger.

Cash, T. F. & Cash, D. W. (1982). Women's use of cosmetics: Psychosocial correlates and consequences. *International Journal of Cosmetic Science, 4,* 1–14.

Cash, T. F., Kehr, J., Polyson, J. & Freeman V. (1977). The role of physical attractiveness in peer attribution of psychological disturbance. *Journal of Consulting and Clinical Psychology, 45,* 987–993.

Casper, R. C., Ekert, E. D., Halmi, K., Goldberg, S. C. & Davis, J. (1980). Bulimia: Its incidence, and clinical importance in patients with anorexia nervosa. *Archives of General Psychiatry, 37,* 1030–1035.

Coll, M., Meyers, M. J. & Stunkard, A. J. (1979). Obesity and food choices in public places. *Archives of General Psychiatry, 36,* 795–797.

Cooley, C. H. (1956). *Human Nature and the Social Order*. Glencoe: Free Press.

Coopersmith, S. (1967). *The Antecedents of Self-Esteem*. San Francisco: W. H. Freeman.

Cotton, N. (1983). The development of self-esteem and self-esteem regulation. In J. E. Mack, & S. L. Ablon (Eds.), *The Development and Sustaining of Self-Esteem in Childhood* (pp 122–150). New York: International Universities Press.

Cottraux, J., Mollard, E. & Defayolle, M. (1982). Behavioral and bodily self concept changes after assertive training. *Acta Psychiatrica Belgica, 82,* 136–146.

Craighead, L. W. (1984). Sequencing of behavior therapy and pharmacotherapy for obesity. *Journal of Consulting and Clinical Psychology, 52,* 190–199.

Crisp, A. H. (1970). Anorexia nervosa, feeding disorder, nervous malnutrition or weight phobia? *World Review of Nutrition, 12,* 452–504.

Crisp, A. H. & Kalucy, R. S. (1974). Aspects of the perceptual disorder in anorexia nervosa. *British Journal of Medical Psychology, 47,* 349–361.

Crisp, A. H. & McGuiness, B. (1976). Jolly fat: Relation between obesity and psychoneurosis in general population. *British Medical Journal, 3,* 7–9.

Crumpton, E., Wine, D. B. & Groot, H. (1966). MMPI profiles of obese men and six other diagnostic categories. *Psychological Reports, 19,* 1110–1115.

Devins, G. M. & Orme, C. M. (1985). Center for Epidemiologic Studies Depression Scale. In D. J. Keyser, & R. C. Sweetland (Eds.), *Test Critiques,* Vol. II. Kansas City, Missouri: Test Corporation of America.

De Vries, H. A. (1968). Immediate and long-term effects of exercise upon resting muscle action potential level. *Journal of Sports Medicine and Physical Fitness, 8,* 1–11.

Donahoe, C. P., Lin, D. H., Kirschenbaum, D. S. & Keesey, R. E. (1984). Metabolic consequences of dieting and exercise in the treatment of obesity. *Journal of Consulting and Clinical Psychology, 52,* 827–836.

Drenick, E. J. (1979). Definition and health consequences of morbid obesity. *Surgical Clinics of North America, 59,* 963–976.

Drewnowski, A. & Yee, D. K. (1987). Men and body image: Are males satisfied with their body weight? *Psychosomatic Medicine, 49,* 626–634.

Dulloo, A. G. & Miller, D. S. (1986). The thermogenic properties of ephedrine/ methylxanthine mixtures: Human studies. *International Journal of Obesity, 10,* 467–481.

Dulloo, A. G. & Miller, D. S. (1987). Aspirin as a promoter of ephedrine-induced thermogenesis: Potential use in the treatment of obesity. *American Journal of Clinical Nutrition, 45,* 564–569.

Eagly, A. H. (1967). Involvement as a determinant of response to favourable and unfavourable information. *Journal of Personality and Social Psychology, 7* (3, pt 2), 1–15.

Elder, G. H. (1969). Appearance and education in marriage mobility. *American Sociological Review, 34,* 519–527.

Epstein, F. H., Francis, T., Hayner, N. S., Johnson, B. C., Kjelsberg, M. O., Napier, J. A., Ostrander, E. D., Payne, M. W. & Dodge, H. J. (1965). Prevalence of chronic diseases and distribution of selected physiologic variables in a total community, Tecumseh, Michigan. *American Journal of Epidemiology, 81,* 307–322.

Ernsberger, P. & Haskew, P. (1987). Health implications of obesity: An alternative view. *Journal of Obesity and Weight Regulation, 6,* 58–81.

Ersek, R. A., Zambrano, J., Surak, G. S. & Denton, D. R. (1986). Suction-assisted lipectomy for correction of 202 figure flaws in 101 patients: Indications, limitations, and applications. *Plastic and Reconstructive Surgery, 78,* 615–626.

Fairburn, C. G. & Cooper, P. J. (1982). Self-induced vomiting and bulimia nervosa: An undetected problem. *British Medical Journal, 284,* 1153–1155.

Fat execs get slimmer paycheck. (1974). *Industry Week, 180,* 21, 24.

Feeling fat in a thin society. (1984). *Glamour Magazine,* February, 198–201, 251–252.

Feinleib, M., Garrison, R. J., Fabsitz, R., Christian, J. C., Hrubec, Z., Borham, N. O., Kannel, N. B., Rosenman, R., Schwartz, J. T. & Wagner, J. O. (1977). The NHLBI twin study of cardiovascular disease risk factors: Methodology and summary of results. *American Journal of Epidemiology, 106,* 284–295.

Ferguson, J. M. & Feighner, J. P. (1987). Fluoxetine-induced weight loss in overweight non-depressed humans. *International Journal of Obesity, 11,* 163–170.

Fitts, W. H. (1972). *The Self-Concept and Psychopathology.* Nashville: Dede Wallace Center.

Fleming, J. S. & Watts, W. A. (1980). The dimensionality of self-esteem: Some results for a college sample. *Journal of Personality and Social Psychology, 39,* 921–929.

Folkins, C. H., Lynch, S. & Gardner, M. M. (1972). Psychological fitness as a function of physical fitness. *Archives of Physical Medicine and Rehabilitation, 53,* 503–508.

Folkins, C. H. & Sime, W. E. (1981). Physical fitness training and mental health. *American Psychologist, 36,* 373–389.

Foreyt, J. P., Goodrick, G. K. & Gotto, A. M. (1981). Limitations of behavioral treatment of obesity: Review and analysis. *Journal of Behavioral Medicine, 4,* 159–174.

Freud, S. (1923). *The Ego and the Id.* In J. Strachey (Ed.) (1961), Standard Edition. London: Hogarth Press.

Garfinkel, P. E. & Garner, D. M. (1982). *Anorexia Nervosa: A Multidimensional Perspective.* New York: Bruner/Mazel.

Garfinkel, P. E. & Garner, D. M. (1984). Perceptions of the body in Anorexia Nervosa. In K. M. Pirke & D. Ploog (Eds.), *The Psychobiology of Anorexia Nervosa* (pp. 136–147). Berlin: Springer.

Garfinkel, P. E., Moldofsky, H., Garner, D. M., Stancer, H. C. & Coscina, D. V. (1978). Body awareness in anorexia nervosa: Disturbances in "body image" and "satiety". *Psychosomatic Medicine, 40,* 487–498.

Garner, D. M. & Garfinkel, P. E. (1981). Body image in anorexia nervosa: Measurement, theory and clinical implications. *International Journal of Psychiatry in Medicine, 11,* 263–284.

Garner, D. M., Garfinkel, P. E., Schwartz, D. & Thompson, M. (1980). Cultural expectations of thinness in women. *Psychological Reports, 47,* 483–491.

Garner, D. M., Garfinkel, P. E., Stancer, H. & Moldofsky, H. (1976). Body image disturbances in anorexia nervosa and obesity. *Psychosomatic Medicine, 38,* 327–336.

Garner, D. M., Olmsted, M. & Polivy, J. (1983). Development and validation of a multidimensional eating disorder inventory for anorexia nervosa and bulimia. *International Journal of Eating Disorders, 2,* 15–34.

Garner, D. M., Rockert, W., Olmsted, M. P., Johnson, C. & Coscina, D. V. (1985). Psychoeducational principles in the treatment of bulimia and anorexia nervosa. In D. M. Garner and P. E. Garfinkel (Eds.), *Handbook of Psychotherapy for Anorexia Nervosa and Bulimia* (pp. 513–572). New York: Guilford Press.

Geissler, C. A., Miller, D. S. & Shah, M. (1987). The daily metabolic rate of the post-obese and the lean. *American Journal of Clinical Nutrition, 45,* 914–920.

Glucksman, M. L. (1972). Psychiatric observations on obesity. *Advances in Psychosomatic Medicine, 7,* 194–216.

Glucksman, M. L. & Hirsch, J. (1968). The response of obese patients to weight reduction: A clinical evaluation of behavior. *Psychosomatic Medicine, 30,* 1–11.

Glucksman, M. L. & Hirsch, J. (1969). The response of obese patients to weight reduction: III. The perception of body size. *Psychosomatic Medicine, 31,* 1–7.

Goldblatt, P. B., Moore, M. E. & Stunkard, A. J. (1965). Social factors in obesity. *Journal of the American Medical Association, 192,* 1039–1044.

Goodman, N., Dornbusch, S. M., Richardson, S. A. & Hastorf, A. H. (1963). Variant reactions to physical disabilities. *American Sociological Review, 28,* 429–435.

Gottheil, E. & Joseph, R. J. (1968). Age, appearance, and schizophrenia. *Archives of General Psychiatry, 19,* 232–238.

Gross, J. & Rosen, J. C. (1988). Bulimia in adolescents: Prevalence and psychosocial correlates. *International Journal of Eating Disorders, 7,* 51–61.

Halmi, K. A., Mason, E., Falk, J. & Stunkard, A. J. (1981). Appetitive behavior after gastric bypass for obesity. *International Journal of Obesity, 5,* 457–464.

Halmi, K. A., Stunkard, A. J. & Mason, E. E. (1980). Emotional responses to weight reduction by three methods: Diet, jejunoileal bypass, and gastric bypass. *American Journal of Clinical Nutrition, 33,* 446–451.

Harris, M. B., Harris, R. J. & Bochner, S. (1982). Fat, four-eyed, and female: Stereotypes of obesity, glasses, and gender. *Journal of Applied Social Psychology, 12,* (6), 503–516.

Hayakawa, S. (1963). *Symbol, Status and Personality.* New York: Brace & World.

Haynes, R. B. (1986). Is weight loss an effective treatment for hypertension? The evidence against. *Canadian Journal of Physiology and Pharmacology, 64,* 825–830.

Health and Welfare Canada (1954). *Canadian Average Weights for Height, Age and Sex.* Nutrition Discussion Paper of the Department of Health and Welfare, Ottawa.

Heatherton, T. (1986). *Restraint and Misattribution: An Analysis of Cognitive Control Mechanisms.* Unpublished Master's thesis, University of Toronto, Canada.

Heatherton, T., Herman, C. P., Polivy, J., King, G. A. & McCree, S. T. (1988). The (mis)measurement of restraint: An analysis of conceptual and psychometric issues. *Journal of Abnormal Psychology, 97,* 19–28.

Herman, C. P. & Mack, D. (1975). Restrained and unrestrained eating. *Journal of Personality, 43,* 647–660.

Herman, C. P. & Polivy, J. (1975). Anxiety, restraint, and eating behavior. *Journal of Abnormal Psychology, 84,* 666–672.

Herman, C. P. & Polivy, J. (1980). Restrained Eating. In A. J. Stunkard (Ed.), *Obesity* (pp. 208–224). Toronto: W. B. Saunders.

Herman, C. P. & Polivy, J. (1984). A boundary model for the regulation of eating. In A. J. Stunkard, & E. Stellar (Eds.), *Eating and Its Disorders* (141–156). New York: Raven.

Hervey, G. R. & Tobin, G. (1983). Luxuskonsumption, diet-induced thermogenesis and brown fat: A critical review. *Clinical Science, 64* 7–18.

Hibscher, J. & Herman, C. P. (1977). Obesity, dieting, and the expression of "obese" characteristics. *Journal of Comparative and Physiological Psychology, 91,* 374–380.

Hilyer, J. & Mitchell, W. (1979). Effect of systematic physical fitness training combined with counselling on the self-concept of college students. *Journal of Counselling Psychology, 26,* 427–436.

Hollingshead, A. B. & Redlich, F. C. (1958). *Social Class and Mental Illness: A Community Study.* New York: Wiley.

Horney, K. (1950). *Neurosis and Human Growth.* New York: Norton.

Hubert, H. B., Feinleib, M., McNamara, P. M. & Castelli, W. P. (1983). Obesity as an independent risk factor for cardiovascular disease: A 26-year follow-up of participants in the Framingham heart study. *Circulation, 67,* 968–977.

Hudson, J. I., Pope, H. G., Wurtman, J., Yurgelun-Todd, D., Mark, S. & Rosenthal, N. E. (1988). Bulimia in obese individuals: Relationship to normal-weight bulimia. *Journal of Nervous and Mental Disease, 176,* 144–152.

Hutchinson, M. G. (1985). *Transforming Body Image.* New York: The Crossing Press.

Jacobovits, C., Halstead, P., Kelley, L., Roe, D. A. & Young, C. M. (1977). Eating habits and nutrient intakes of college women over a thirty year period. *Journal of the American Dietetic Association, 71,* 405–411.

Janis, I. L. & Field, P. B. (1959). Sex differences in personality factors related to persuasibility. In C. I. Hovland, & I. L. Janis (Eds.), *Personality and Persuasibility,* (pp. 55–68). New Haven: Yale University Press.

Jourard, S. M. & Secord, P. R. (1955). Body-cathexis and the ideal female figure. *Journal of Abnormal and Social Psychology, 50,* 243–246.

Kalucy, R. S., Gilchrist, P. N., McFarlane, C. M. & McFarlane, A. C. (1985). The evolution of a multidisciplinary orientation. In D. M. Garner & P. E. Garfinkel (Eds.), *Handbook of Psychotherapy for Anorexia Nervosa and Bulimia* (pp. 458–487). New York: Guilford.

Kaplan, S. L., Busner, J. & Pollack, S. (1988). Perceived weight, actual weight, and depressive symptoms in a general adolescent sample. *International Journal of Eating Disorders, 7,* 107–113.

Kaplan, H. I. & Kaplan, H. S. (1957). The psychosomatic concept of obesity. *Journal of Nervous and Mental Disorders, 125,* 181–201.

Kaufman, N. A. (1986). Gastric balloon treatment: Past, present, future. In E. M. Beery, S. H. Blondheim, H. E. Eliahou & E. Shafrir (Eds.), *Recent Advances in Obesity Research: V,* (pp. 373–374). London: John Libbey.

Keefe, P. H., Wyshogrod, D., Weinberger, E. & Agras, W. S. (1984). Binge eating and outcome of behavioral treatment for obesity: A preliminary report. *Behavior Research and Therapy, 22,* 319–321.

Keesey, R. E. (1980). A set-point analysis of the regulation of body weight. In A. J. Stunkard (Ed.), *Obesity* (pp. 144–165). Toronto: W. B. Saunders.

Keesey, R. E. (1986). A set-point theory of obesity. In K. D. Brownell & J. P. Foreyt (Eds.), *Handbook of Eating Disorders: Physiology, Psychology, & Treatment of Obesity, Anorexia and Bulimia* (pp. 63–87). New York: Basic Books.

Keys, A., Brozek, J., Henschel, A., Mickelson, O. & Taylor, H. L. (1950). *The Biology of Human Starvation.* Minneapolis: University of Minneapolis.

Kissebah, A. H., Vydelingum, N., Murray, R., Evans, D. J., Harty, A. J., Kalkhoff, R. K. & Adams, P. W. (1982). Relation of body fat distribution to metabolic complications of obesity. *Journal of Clinical Endocrinology and Metabolism, 54,* 254–260.

Kissileff, K. S., Jordan, H. A. & Levitz, L. S. (1978). Eating habits of obese and normal weight humans. *International Journal of Obesity, 2,* 379.

Kohut, H. (1977). *The Restoration of the Self.* New York: International Universities Press.

Krotkiewski, M. L., Bjorntorp, P., Sjostrom, L. & Smith, U. (1983). Impact of obesity on metabolism in men and women. *Journal of Clinical Investigation, 72,* 115–116.

Laessle, R. G., Kittl, S., Fichter, M. M., Wittchen H. U. & Pirke, K. M. (1987). Major affective disorder in Anorexia Nervosa and Bulimia: A descriptive diagnostic study. *British Journal of Psychiatry, 151,* 785–789.

Lapidus, L., Gengtsson, C., Larrson, B., Pennert, K., Rybo, E. & Sjostrom, L. (1984). Distribution of adipose tissue and risk of cardiovascular disease and death. A 12-year follow-up of participants in the population study of women in Gothenburg, Sweden. *British Medical Journal, 289,* 1257–1261.

Larkin, J. E. & Pines, H. A. (1979). No fat persons need apply. *Sociology of Work and Occupations, 63* 312–327.

Larrson, B., Svardsudd, K., Welin, L., Wilhelmsen, L., Bjorntorp, P. & Tibblin, G. (1984). Abdominal adipose tissue distribution, obesity, and risk of cardiovascular disease and death: A thirteen year follow-up of participants in the study of men born in 1913. *British Medical Journal, 288,* 1401–1404.

Leiter, L. A. (1985). Obesity: Overview of pathogenesis and treatment. *Canadian Journal of Physiology and Pharmacology, 64,* 814–817.

Lerner, R. M., Karabenick, S. A. & Stuart, J. L. (1973). Relations among physical attractiveness, body attitudes, and self-concept in male and female college students. *Journal of Psychology, 85,* 119–129.

Lerner, R. M., Orlos, J. B. & Knapp, J. R. (1976). Physical attractiveness, physical effectiveness and self concept in late adolescents. *Adolescence, 11,* 313–326.

Levitz, L. S. & Stunkard, A. J. (1974). A therapeutic coalition for obesity: Behavior modification and patient self-help. *American Journal of Psychiatry, 131,* 423–427.

Lew, E. A. & Garfinkel, L. (1979). Variations in mortality by weight among 750,000 men and women. *Journal of Chronic Disease, 32,* 563–576.

Linet, O. I. & Metzler, C. M. (1981). Emotional status during weight reduction programs. *Journal of Clinical Psychiatry, 42,* 228–232.

Lowe, C. (1961). The self-concept: Fact or artifact? *Psychological Bulletin, 58,* 325–336.

Lowe, M. R. (1984) Dietary concern, weight fluctuation and weight status: Further explorations of the Restraint Scale. *Behavior Research and Therapy, 22,* 234–248.

MacMahon, S., Cutler, J., Brittain, E. & Higgins, M. (1987). Obesity and hypertension: epidemiological and clinical issues. *European Heart Journal, 8,* 57–70.

Maddox, G. L., Black, K. & Liederman, V. (1968). Overweight as social deviance and disability. *Journal of Health and Social Behavior, 9,* 287–298.

Mahoney, E. R. (1974). Body-cathexis and self-esteem: The importance of subjective importance. *Journal of Psychology, 88,* 27–30.

Mahoney, M. J. (1975). The obese eating style: Bites, beliefs and behavior modification. *Addictive Behaviors, 1,* 47–53.

Manson, J. E., Stampfer, M. J., Hennekens, C. H. & Willett, W. C. (1987). Body weight and longevity: A reassessment. *Journal of the American Medical Association, 257,* 353–358.

Marston, A. R. & Criss, J. (1984). Maintenance of successful weight loss: Incidence and predictors. *International Journal of Obesity, 8,* 435–439.

Martinek, T. J., Cheffers, J. T. & Zaichowsky, L. D. (1978). Physical activity, motor development and self-concept: Race and age differences. *Perceptual and Motor Skills, 46,* 147–154.

Maslow, A. (1954). *Motivation and Personality.* New York: Harper.

Mayer, J. (1966). Obesity: Progress and remaining ignorance. In F. J. Ingelfinger, & A. S. Relman (Eds.), *Controversy in Internal Medicine* (pp. 453–463). Philadelphia: W. B. Saunders.

Mazur, A. (1986). U. S. trends in feminine beauty and overadaptation. *Journal of Sex Research, 22,* 281–303.

McCrea, C. W., Summerfield, A. B. & Rosen, B. (1982). Body image: A selective review of existing measurement techniques. *British Journal of Medical Psychology, 55,* 225–233.

McFarland, R. J., Gazet, J. C. & Pilkington, T. R. E. (1985). A 13-year review of jejunoileal bypass. *British Journal of Surgery, 72,* 81–83.

McFarland, R. J., Grundy, A., Gazet, J. C. & Pilkington, T. R. E. (1987). The intragastric balloon: A novel idea proved ineffective. *British Journal of Surgery, 74,* 137–139.

McGowan, R. W., Jarman, B. O. & Pederson, D. M. (1974). Effects of a competitive endurance training program on self-concept and peer approval. *Journal of Psychology, 86,* 57–60.

McReynolds, W. T. (1982). Toward a psychology of obesity: Review of research on the role of personality and level of adjustment. *International Journal of Eating Disorders, 2,* 37–57.

Meisenhelder, J. B. (1985). Self esteem: A closer look at clinical interventions. *International Journal of Nursing Studies, 22,* 127–135.

Miller, D. S. (1982). Factors affecting energy expenditure. *Proceedings of the Nutrition Society, 41,* 193–202.

Moore, M. E., Stunkard, A. J. & Srole, L. (1962). Obesity, social class and mental illness. *Journal of the American Medical Association, 181,* 962–966.

Morgan, W. P., Roberts, J. A., Brand, F. R. & Feinerman, A. D. (1970). Psychological effects of chronic physical activity. *Medicine and Science in Sports, 2,* 213–217.

Mrosovsky, N. & Powley, T. L. (1977). Set points for body weight and fat. *Behavioral Biology, 20,* 205–223.

Musa, K. E. & Roach, M. E. (1973). Adolescent appearance and self-concept. *Adolescence, 8,* 385–394.

National Institutes of Health Consensus Development Conference Statement. (1985). Health implications of obesity. *Annals of Internal Medicine, 103,* 147–151.

Neumann, R. O. (1902). Experimentalle Beitrage zur Lehre von dem taglichen Nahrungsbedarf des Menschen unter besonderer Berucksichtigung der notwendigen Eiweissmenge. *Archiv fur Hygiene, 45,* 1–87.

Newsholme, E. A. (1982). The interrelationship between metabolic regulation, weight control and obesity. *Proceedings of the Nutrition Society, 41,* 183–191.

Noles, S. W., Cash, T. F. & Winstead, B.A. (1985). Body image, physical attractiveness, and depression. *Journal of Consulting and Clinical Psychology, 53,* 88–94.

Norusis, M. J. (1988). *SPSS/PC+ Advanced Statistics V2.0.* Chicago: SPSS Inc.

Nutzinger, D. O., Cayiroglu, S., Sachs, G. & Zapotoczky, H. G. (1985). Emotional problems during weight reduction: Advantages of a combined behavior therapy and antidepressive drug therapy for obesity. *Journal of Behavior Therapy and Experimental Psychiatry, 16,* 217–221.

Orbach, S. (1978). *Fat is a Feminist Issue.* New York: Paddington Press.

Pacy, P. J., Webster, J. & Garrow, J. S. (1986). Exercise and obesity. *Sports Medicine, 3,* 89–113.

Pearlson, G. D., Flournoy, L. H., Simonson, M. & Slavney, P. R. (1981). Body image in obese adults. *Psychological Medicine, 11,* 147–154.

Pliner, P., Chaiken, S. & Flett, G. L. (1987). Concern with body weight and physical appearance over the lifespan. Unpublished paper.

Polivy, J., Heatherton, T. F. & Herman, C. P. (1988). Self-esteem, restraint, and eating behavior. *Journal of Abnormal Psychology, 85,* 601–606.

Polivy, J., & Herman, C. P. (1976). Effects of alcohol on eating behavior: Influences of mood and perceived intoxication. *Journal of Abnormal Psychology, 85,* 601–606.

Polivy, J. & Herman, C. P. (1983). *Breaking the Diet Habit.* New York: Basic Books.

Polivy, J. & Herman, C. P. (1985). Dieting and bingeing: A causal analysis. *American Psychologist, 40,* 193–201.

Polivy, J. & Herman, C. P. (1987). Diagnosis and treatment of normal eating. *Journal of Consulting and Clinical Psychology, 55,* 635–644.

Polivy, J., Herman, C. P., Olmsted, M. P. & Jazwinski, C. M. (1984). Restraint and binge eating. In R. C. Hawkins, W. Fremouw, & P. F. Clement (Eds.), *The Binge-Purge Syndrome: Diagnosis, Treatment, and Research* (pp. 104–122). New York: Springer.

Prather, R. C. & Williamson, D. A. (1988). Psychopathology associated with bulimia, binge eating, and obesity. *International Journal of Eating Disorders, 7,* 177–184.

Pudel, V. E. (1975). Psychological observations on experimental feeding in the obese. In Howard, A. (Ed.) *Recent Advances in Obesity Research* (pp. 66–74). London: Newman.

Pyle, R. L., Mitchell, J. E. & Eckert, E. D. (1981). Bulimia: A report of 34 cases. *Journal of Clinical Psychiatry, 42,* 60–64.

Radloff, L. S. (1977). The CES-D Scale: A new self-report depression scale for research in the general population. *Applied Psychological Measurement, 1,* 385–401.

Ravussin, E., Lillioja, S., Knowler, W. C., Christen, L., Freymond, D., Abbott, W. G. H., Boyce, V., Howard, B. V. & Bogardus, C. (1988). Reduced rate of energy expenditure as a risk factor for body-weight gain. *New England Journal of Medicine, 318,* 467–472.

Richardson, S. A., Goodman, N., Hastorf, A. H. & Dornbusch, S. M. (1961). Cultural uniformity in reaction to physical disabilities. *American Social Review, 26,* 241–247.

Roberts, N. (1985). *Breaking All the Rules.* New York: Penguin.

Robson, P. J. (1988). Self-esteem—a psychiatric view. *British Journal of Psychiatry, 153,* 6–15.

Rosen, J. C., Gross, J. & Vara, L. (1987). Psychological adjustment of adolescents attempting to lose or gain weight. *Journal of Consulting and Clinical Psychology, 55,* 742–747.

Rosen, G. M. & Ross, A. O. (1968). Relationship of body image to self-concept. *Journal of Consulting and Clinical Psychology, 32,* 100.

Rosenberg, M. (1965). *Society and the Adolescent Self-Image.* Princeton University Press.

Rosenberg, M. (1979). *Conceiving the Self.* New York: Basic Books.

Rosenberg, M. (1981). The self-concept: Social product and social force. In M. Rosenberg, & R. H. Turner (Eds.), *Social Psychology: Sociological Perspective* (pp. 593–624). New York: Basic Books.

Rossner, S. (1984). Ideal body weight—for whom? *Acta Medica Scandinavia, 216,* 241–242.

Rossner, S. & Bjorvell, H. (1987). Early and late effects of weight loss on lipoprotein, metabolism in severe obesity. *Atherosclerosis, 64,* 125–130.

Roth, G. (1984). *Breaking Free From Compulsive Eating.* New York: Signet.

Rothwell, N. J. & Stock, M. J. (1983). Luxuskonsumption, diet-induced thermogenesis and brown fat: The case in favour. *Clinical Science, 64,* 19–23.

Ruderman, A. J. (1983). The Restraint Scale: A psychometric investigation. *Behavior Research and Therapy, 21,* 258–283.

Sanford, L. T. & Donovan, M. E. (1985). *Women and Self-Esteem.* New York: Penguin.

Sankowsky, M. H. (1981). The effect of a treatment based on the use of guided visuo-kinesthetic imagery on the alteration of negative body-cathexis in women. Unpublished doctoral dissertation, Boston University School of Education.

Schachter, S. (1971). Some extraordinary facts about obese humans and rats. *American Psychologist, 26,* 129–145.

Schacter, S. (1981). Self-treatment of smoking and obesity. *Canadian Journal of Public Health, 72,* 401–406.

Schlichting, P., Hoilund-Carlsen, P. F. & Quaade, F. (1981). Comparison of self-reported height and weight with controlled height and weight in women and men. *International Journal of Obesity, 5,* 67–76.

Sclafani, A. (1984). Animal models of obesity: A classification and characterization. *International Journal of Obesity, 8,* 491–508.

Secord, P. F. & Jourard, S. M. (1953). The appraisal of body-cathexis: Body cathexis and the self. *Journal of Consulting Psychology, 17,* 343–347.

Shavelson, R. J. & Bolus, R. (1982). Self-concept: The interplay of theory and methods. *Journal of Educational Psychology, 74,* 3–17.

Shipman, W. G. & Sohlkah, N. (1967). Body image distortion in obese women. Paper presented at the National Meeting of the American Psychosomatic Society, April.

Silverstone, J. T. (1968). Psychological aspects of obesity. *Proceedings of the Royal Society of Medicine, 61,* 371–375.

Simopoulos, A. P. & Van Itallie, T. B. (1984). Body weight, health and longevity. *Annals of Internal Medicine, 100,* 285–295.

Sims, E. A., Danforth, E., Horton, E. S., Bray, G. A., Glennon, J. A. & Salans, L. B. (1973). Endocrine and metabolic effects of experimental obesity in man. *Recent Progress in Hormonal Research, 29,* 457–496.

Slade, P. D. & Russell, G. F. M. (1973). Experimental investigations of bodily perception in anorexia nervosa and obesity. *Psychotherapy and Psychosomatics, 22,* 359–363.

Smoller, J. W., Wadden, T. A. & Stunkard, A. J. (1987). Dieting and Depression: A critical review. *Journal of Psychosomatic Research, 31,* 429–440.

Snow, J. & Harris, M. R. (1985). Maintenance of weight loss: Behavioral and attitudinal correlates. *Journal of Obesity and Weight Regulation, 4,* 234–257.

Solow, C., Silverfarb, P. M. & Swift, K. (1974). Psychosocial effects of intestinal bypass surgery for severe obesity. *New England Journal of Medicine, 290,* 300–304.

Staffieri, J. R. (1967). A study of social stereotype of body image in children. *Journal of Personal and Social Psychology, 7,* 101–104.

Stalonas, P. M., Perri, M. G. & Kerzner, A. B. (1984). Do behavioral treatments of obesity last? A five-year follow-up investigation. *Addictive Behaviors, 9,* 175–183.

Stewart, A. L. & Brobek, R. H. (1983). Effects of being overweight. *American Journal of Public Health, 73,* 171–178.

Stunkard, A. J. (1957). The dieting depression: Untoward emotional responses to weight reduction. *American Journal of Medicine, 23,* 77–86.

Stunkard, A. J. (1958). The results of treatment for obesity. *New York State Journal of Medicine, 58,* 79–87.

Stunkard, A. J. (1976). *The Pain of Obesity.* Bull: Palo Alto.

Stunkard, A. J. (1984). The current status of treatment of obesity in adults. In Stunkard, A. J. & Stellar E. (Eds.), *Eating and its Disorders* (pp. 157–173). New York: Raven.

Stunkard, A. J. (1986). The control of obesity: Social and community perspectives. In K. D. Brownell, & J. P. Foreyt (Eds.), *Handbook of Eating Disorders: Physiology, Psychology, and Treatment of Obesity, Anorexia, and Bulimia* (pp. 213–228). New York: Basic Books.

Stunkard, A. J. & Burt, V. (1967). Obesity and body image: II. Age at onset of disturbances in the body image. *American Journal of Psychiatry, 123,* 1443–1447.

Stunkard, A. J., Coll, M., Lindquist, S. & Meyers, A. (1980). Obesity and Eating Style. *Archives of General Psychiatry, 37,* 1127–1129.

Stunkard, A. J., Foch, T. T. & Hrubec, Z. (1986). A twin study of human obesity. *Journal of the American Medical Association, 256,* 51–54.

Stunkard, A. J. & Mendelson, M. (1961). Disturbances in body image of some obese persons. *Journal of the American Dietetic Association, 38,* 328–331.

Stunkard, A. J. & Mendelson, M. (1967). Obesity and body image: I. Characteristics of disturbances in the body image of some obese persons. *American Journal of Psychiatry, 123,* 1296–1300.

Stunkard, A. J. & Messick, S. (1985). The Three-Factor Eating Questionnaire to measure restraint, disinhibition and hunger. *Journal of Psychosomatic Research, 29,* 71–83.

Stunkard, A. J. & Penick, S. B. (1979). Behavior modification in the treatment of obesity. *Archives of General Psychiatry, 36,* 801–806.

Stunkard, A. J. & Rush, J. (1974). Dieting and depression. *Annals of Internal Medicine, 81,* 526–533.

Stunkard, A. J., Sorenson, T. I. A., Hanis, C., Teasdale, T. W., Chakraborty, R., Schull, W. J. & Schulsinger, F. (1986). An adoption study of human obesity. *New England Journal of Medicine, 314,* 193–198.

Stunkard, A. J., Stinnet, J. L. & Smoller, J. W. (1986). Psychological and social aspects of the surgical treatment of obesity. *American Journal of Psychiatry, 143,* 417–429.

Sullivan, A. C. (1986). Drug treatment of obesity: A perspective. In E. M. Berry, S. H. Blondheim, H. E. Eliahou, & E. Shafrir (Eds.), *Recent Advances in Obesity Research: V.* (pp. 293–299). London: John Libbey.

Sullivan, H. S. (1953). *The Interpersonal Theory of Psychiatry.* New York: Norton.

Taylor, C. B., Ferguson, J. M. & Reading, J. C. (1978). Gradual weight loss and depression. *Behavior Therapy, 9,* 622–625.

Telch, C. F., Agras, W. S. & Rossiter, E. M. (1988). Binge eating increases with increasing adiposity. *International Journal of Eating Disorders, 7,* 115–119.

Traub, A. C. & Orbach, J. (1964). Psychophysical studies of body image. *Archives of General Psychiatry, 11,* 53–66.

Van Itallie, T. B. & Yang, M. (1984). Cardiac dysfunction in obese dieters: A potentially lethal complication of rapid, massive weight loss. *American Journal of Clinical Nutrition, 39,* 695–702.

van Strien, T. & Bergers, G. P. A. (1988). Overeating and sex-role orientation in women. *International Journal of Eating Disorders, 7,* 89–99.

Volkmar, F. R., Stunkard, A. J., Woolston, J. & Bailey, B. A. (1981). High attrition rates in commercial weight loss programs. *Archives of Internal Medicine, 141,* 426–428.

Wadden, T. A. & Stunkard, A. J. (1985). Social and psychological consequences of obesity. *Annals of Internal Medicine, 103,* 1062–1067.

Wadden, T., Stunkard, A. J. & Smoller, J. (1986). Dieting and depression: A methodological study. *Journal of Consulting and Clinical Psychology, 6,* 869–871.

Watkins, D. A. & Parks, J. L. (1972). The role of subjective importance in self-evaluation. *Australia Journal of Psychology, 24,* 209–210.

Weissman, M. M. & Bothwell, S. (1976). Assessment of social adjustment by patient self-report. *Archives of General Psychiatry, 33,* 1111–1115.

Weissman, M. M., Prusoff, B. A., Thompson, W. D., Harding, P. S. & Meyers, J. K. (1978). Social adjustment by self-report in a community sample and in psychiatric outpatients. *Journal of Nervous and Mental Disease, 166,* 317–326.

Wells, E. W. & Marwell, G. (1976). *Self Esteem—Its Conceptualization and Measurement.* London: Sage.

White, R. W. (1964). *The Abnormal Personality.* New York: Ronald.

Wing, R. R. & Jeffery, R. W. (1979). Outpatient treatment of obesity: A comparison of methodology and clinical results. *International Journal of Obesity, 3,* 261–279.

Wing, R. R., Epstein, L. H., Marcus, M. D. & Kupfer, D. J. (1984). Mood changes in behavioral weight loss programs. *Journal of Psychosomatic Research, 28,* 189–196.

Wooley, S. C. & Kearney-Cooke, A. (1986). Intensive treatment of bulimia and body image disturbance. In K. Brownell & J. Foreyt (Eds.), *Handbook of Eating Disorders: Physiology, Psychology, and the Treatment of Obesity, Anorexia, and Bulimia* (pp. 476–502). New York: Basic Books.

Wooley, S. C. & Wooley, O. W. (1979). Obesity and women I: A closer look at the facts. *Women's Studies International Quarterly, 2,* 69–79.

Wooley, S. C. & Wooley, O. W. (1984). Should obesity be treated at all? In A. J. Stunkard & E. St llar (Eds.), *Eating and Its Disorders.* New York: Raven Press.

Wooley, S. C., Wooley, O. W. & Dyrenforth, S. R. (1979). Theoretical, practical, and social issues in behavioral treatments of obesity. *Journal of Applied Behavioral Analysis, 12,* 3–25.

Wylie, R. C. (1979). *The Self-Concept.* Lincoln: University of Nebraska Press.

Yager, J., Kurtzman, F., Landsverk, J. & Wiesmeier, E. (1988). Behaviors and attitudes related to eating disorders in homosexual male college students. *American Journal of Psychiatry, 145,* 495–497.

Young, L. M. & Powell, B. (1985). The effects of obesity on the clinical judgments of mental health professionals. *Journal of Health and Social Behavior, 26,* 233–246.

Ziller, R. C. (1973). *The Social Self.* New York: Pergamon Press.

Index